# TYPE 1

## DIABETES

## COOKBOOK

Complete guide for healthy living by balancing your blood sugar

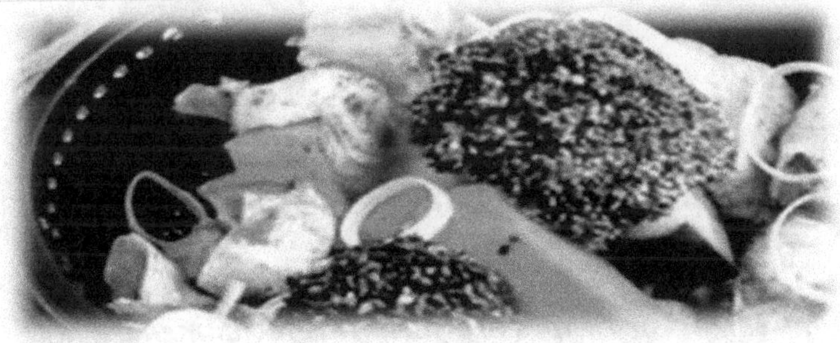

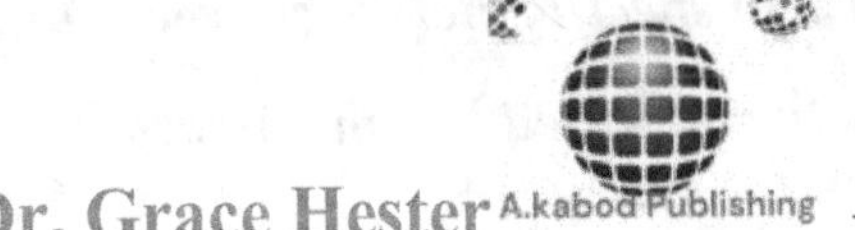

Dr. Grace Hester A.kabod Publishing

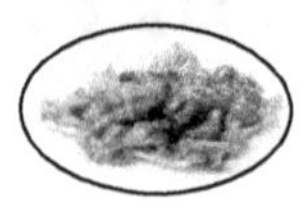 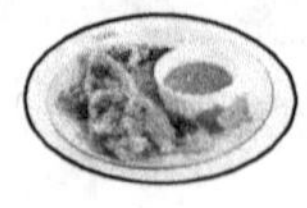 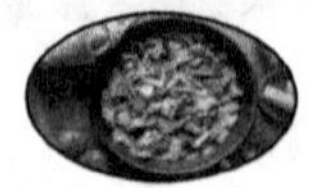

# Copyright Page



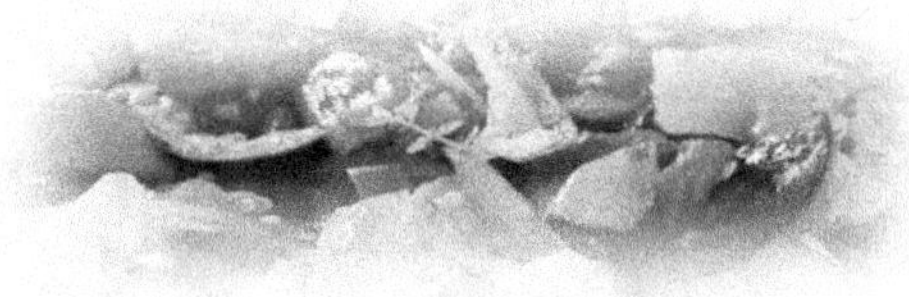

*Disclaimer: The recipes contained in this cookbook are intended for personal use and enjoyment. The author and publisher are not responsible for any health issues or allergic reactions that may arise from the use of the ingredients or recipes provided. It is recommended that individuals with specific dietary concerns or restrictions consult a qualified healthcare professional.*

# DR. GRACE HESTER

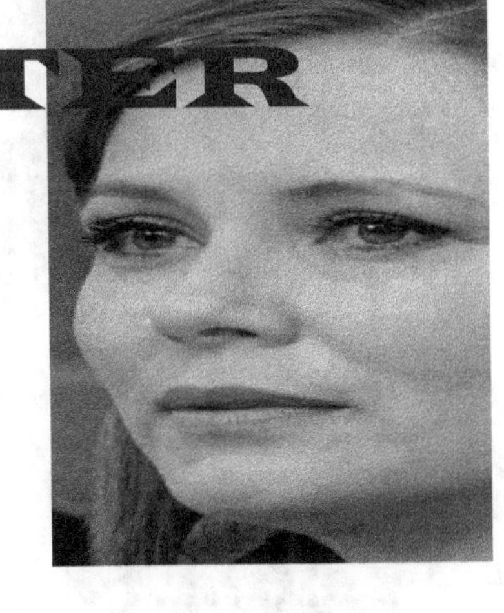

*Dr. Grace Hester stands at the intersection of health, passion, and culinary excellence. A distinguished medical professional and accomplished nutritionist, she seamlessly weaves together her expertise to create a holistic approach to well-being.*

*Dr. Hester earned her medical degree from the renowned Johns Hopkins School of Medicine, consistently ranked among the top medical schools globally. Her commitment to advancing healthcare led her to prestigious positions at the Mayo Clinic, where she honed her skills in internal medicine. Driven by a desire to explore the profound connection between nutrition and overall health, she furthered her education at the Culinary Institute of America.*

*With a deep understanding of both medicine and nutrition, Dr. Hester embarked on a mission to inspire others to embrace a healthier lifestyle. Her culinary journey– led to the creation of a series of cookbooks that blend the art of cooking with the science of nutrition. Each recipe is a testament to her commitment to flavor, nourishment, and well-being.*

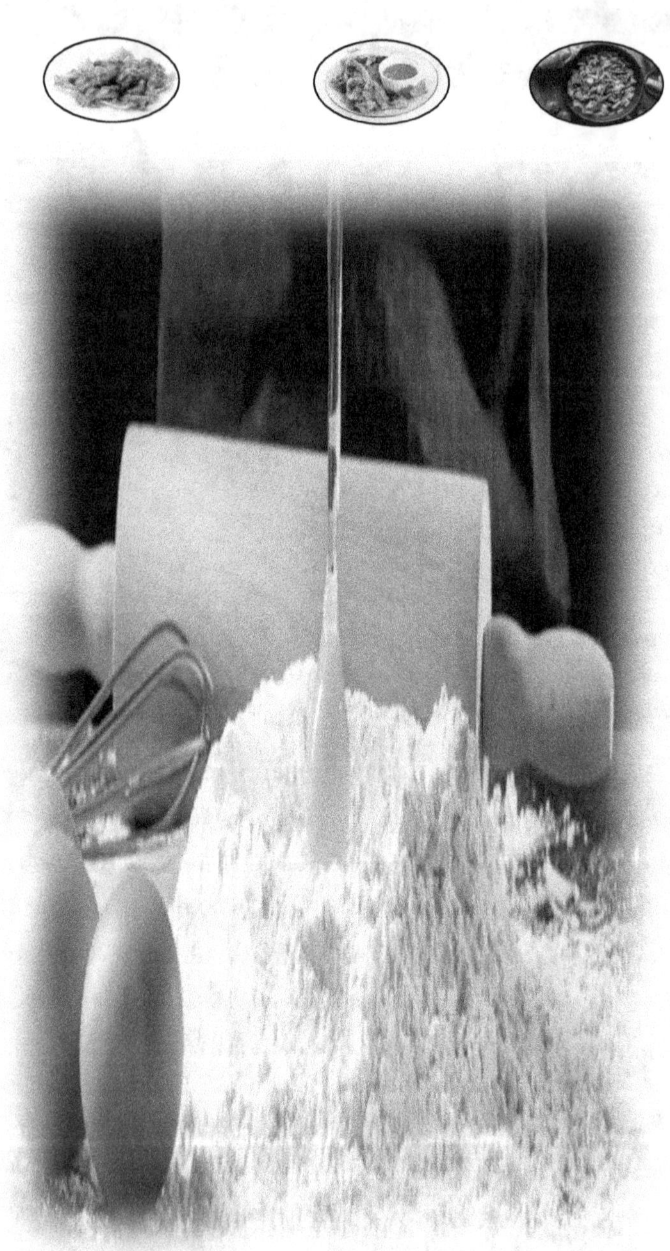

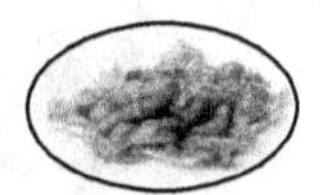 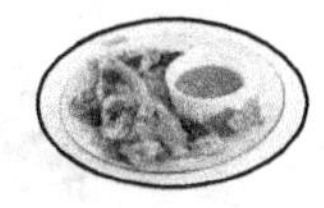 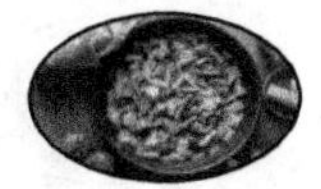

# TABLE OF CONTENT

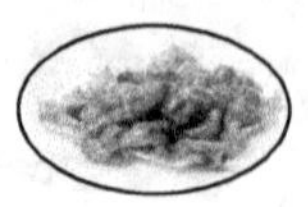
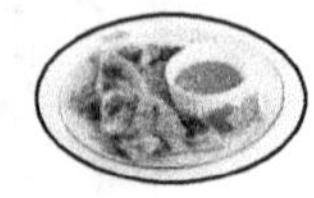
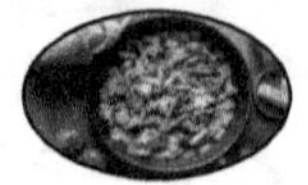



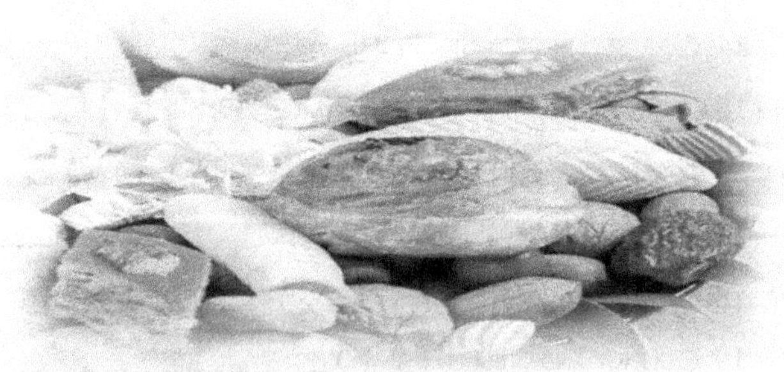

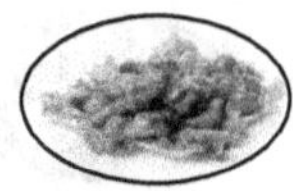 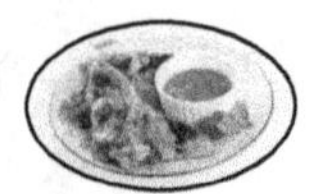 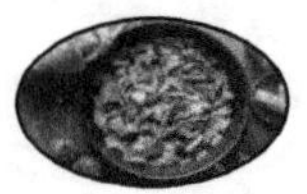

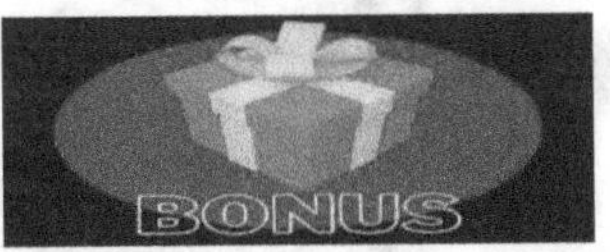

# SCAN THE QR CODE TO GET YOUR FREE HOME MADE GREEN SMOOTHIE RECIPE BOOK

## BONUS 1

Your 20 days meal planner is attached at the end of the book.  Enjoy!

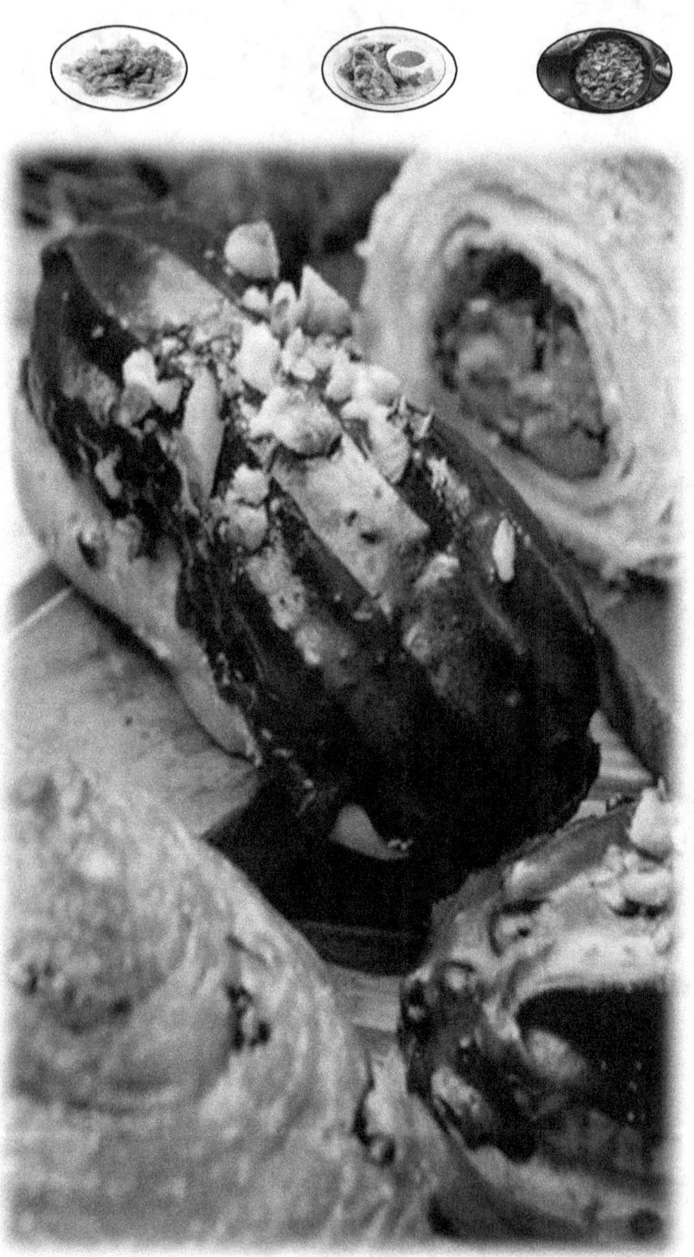

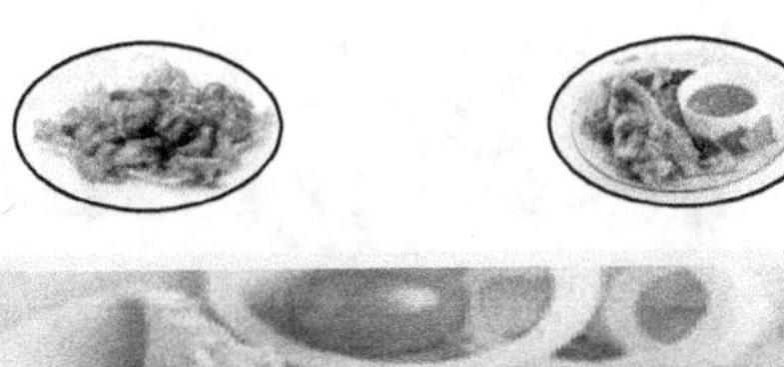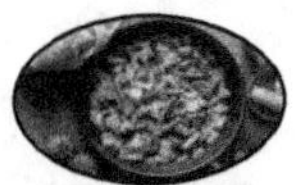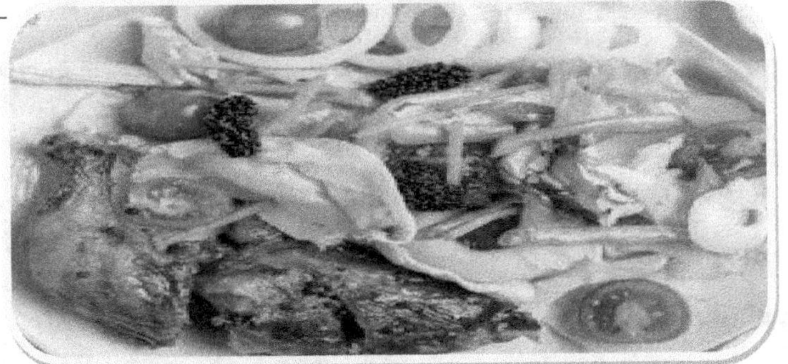

# INTRODUCTION–

## A Journey to Wellness

In the quiet suburbs of a bustling city, lived Sarah, a vibrant young woman navigating life with a determined spirit. Little did she know, her world was about to change when she received a Type 1 diabetes diagnosis. The initial shock and uncertainty swept through her, leaving behind a trail of questions about her future and well-being.

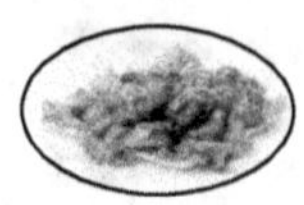 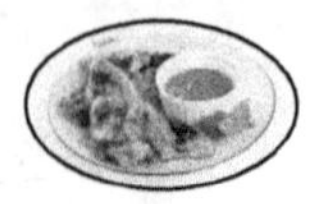 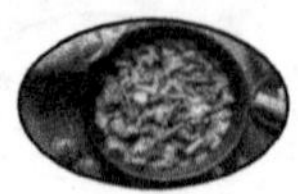

Faced with the challenge of managing her blood sugar levels, Sarah embarked on a journey to discover a balanced and wholesome approach to her new reality. It was during this time that she realized the transformative power of mindful nutrition, discovering that the right foods could be both delicious and diabetes-friendly.

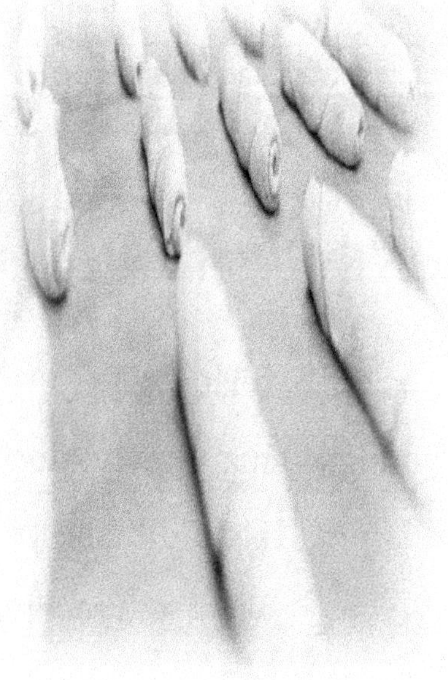

As Sarah navigated through the labyrinth of dietary adjustments, she encountered a myriad of flavors, textures, and culinary delights that not only satisfied her taste buds but also helped stabilize her blood sugar levels. It was this revelation that inspired the creation of the "Type 1 Diabetes Cookbook: A Complete Guide for Healthy Living by Balancing Your Blood Sugar."

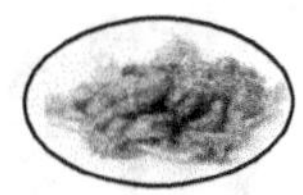 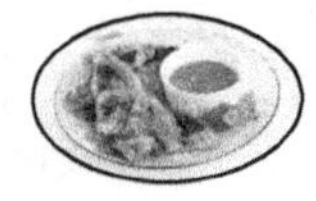 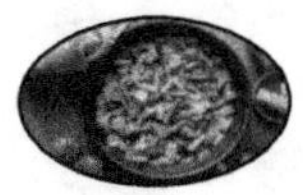

This cookbook isn't just a compilation of recipes; it's a lifeline for those, like Sarah, seeking a way to embrace a healthy lifestyle while managing Type 1 diabetes. Each recipe is crafted with precision and care, combining wholesome ingredients to create dishes that not only nourish the body but also bring joy to the table.

In the pages that follow, you'll find a collection of recipes that go beyond the ordinary, offering a diverse array of flavors that cater to different tastes and preferences. From hearty main courses to refreshing salads, each dish is designed to help maintain blood sugar levels while embracing the joy of eating.

Sarah's journey becomes a guiding light for all those facing the challenges of Type 1 diabetes. Through the carefully curated recipes in this book, she discovered that food could be a source of empowerment, enabling her to live a full and vibrant life. It is our hope that as you embark on your own culinary adventure with these recipes, you too will find not only nourishment for your body but also a renewed sense of vitality and well-being.

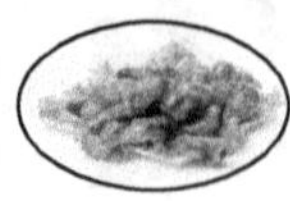 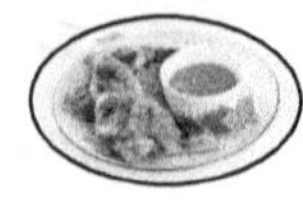 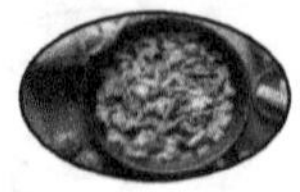

Welcome to the "Type 1 Diabetes Cookbook," where each recipe is a step toward a healthier, more balanced life. May these dishes inspire and empower you on your journey to wellness.

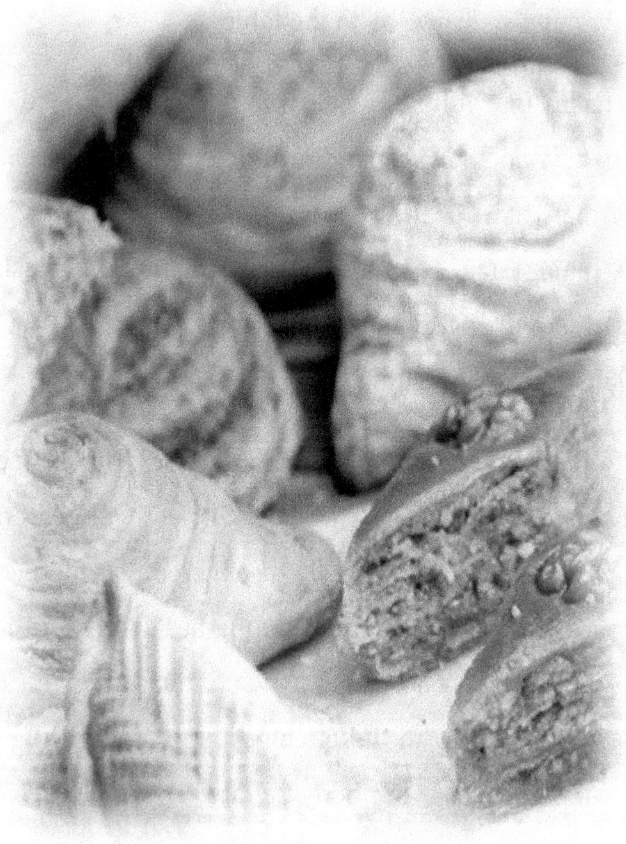

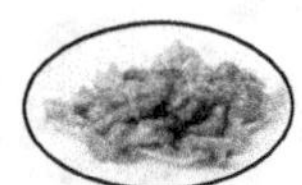 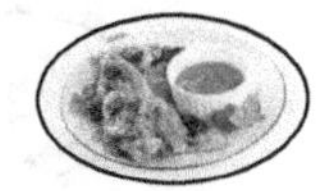 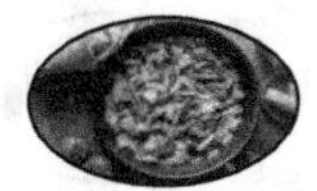



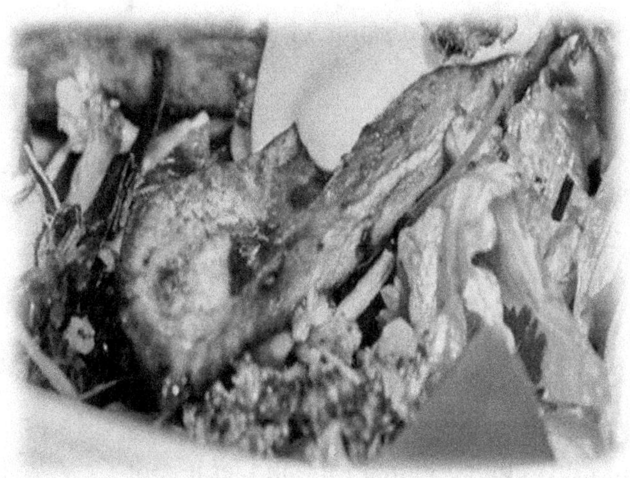

**Ingredients:**

- 1 cup quinoa, rinsed

- 2 cups water

- 1 cup cherry tomatoes, halved

- 1 cucumber, diced

- 1/2 red onion, finely chopped–

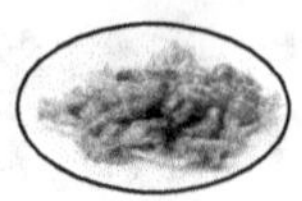 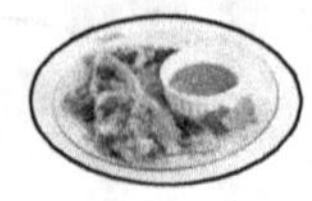 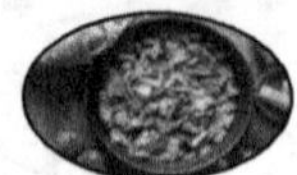

- 1/4 cup feta cheese, crumbled

- 2 tablespoons olive oil

- 1 tablespoon balsamic vinegar

- Salt and pepper to taste

**Instructions:**

1. In a saucepan, combine quinoa and water. Bring to a boil, then reduce heat, cover, and simmer for 15 minutes or until quinoa is cooked.

2. Fluff quinoa with a fork and let it cool.

3. In a large bowl, mix quinoa, cherry tomatoes, cucumber, red onion, and feta cheese.

4. In a small bowl, whisk together olive oil, balsamic vinegar, salt, and pepper.

5. Drizzle the dressing over the salad and toss gently to combine.

6. Serve chilled.–

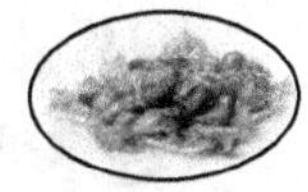 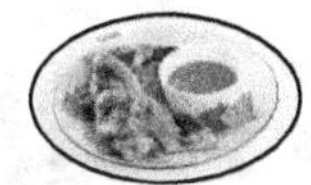 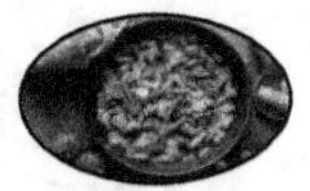

# Recipe 2: Grilled Chicken Breast

**Ingredients:**

- 4 boneless, skinless chicken breasts

- 2 tablespoons olive oil

- 1 teaspoon garlic powder

- 1 teaspoon paprika

- 1 teaspoon dried oregano

- Salt and pepper to taste

**Instructions:**

1. Preheat the grill to medium-high heat.

2. In a small bowl, mix olive oil, garlic powder, paprika, oregano, salt, and pepper to create a marinade.

3. Brush the marinade over the chicken breasts.

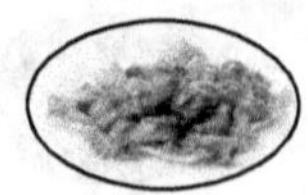 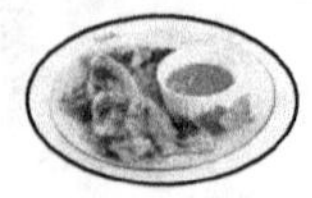 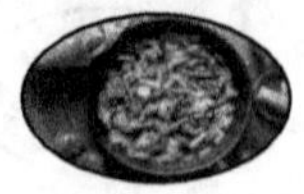

4.  Grill the chicken for 6-8 minutes per side or until no longer pink in the center.

5.  Let it rest for a few minutes before slicing.

6.  Serve with a side of roasted vegetables.

## Recipe 3: Zucchini Noodles with Pesto

**Ingredients:**

- 4 zucchinis, spiralized

- 1 cup cherry tomatoes, sliced

- 1/2 cup fresh basil leaves

- 1/4 cup pine nuts

- 1/2 cup Parmesan cheese, grated

- 2 cloves garlic

- 1/2 cup olive oil

- Salt and pepper to taste

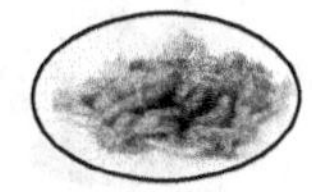 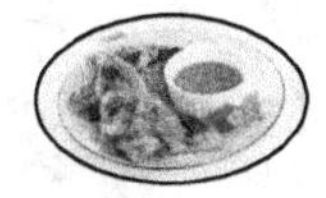 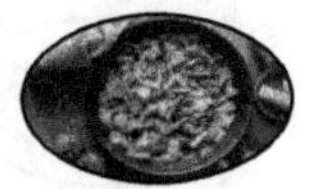

**Instructions:**

1. In a blender, combine basil, pine nuts, Parmesan, garlic, and olive oil. Blend until smooth.

2. In a pan, sauté zucchini noodles until tender.

3. Add cherry tomatoes and cook for an additional 2 minutes.

4. Toss the zucchini and tomatoes with the pesto sauce.

5. Season with salt and pepper.

6. Serve warm.

## Recipe 4: Salmon with Lemon-Dill Sauce

**Ingredients:**

- 4 salmon fillets
- 2 tablespoons olive oil–

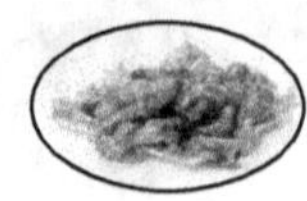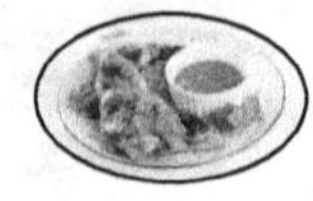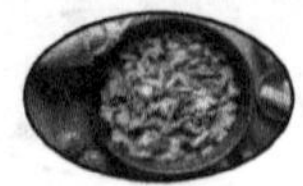

- 1 teaspoon dried dill

- Juice of 1 lemon

- Salt and pepper to taste

## Instructions:

1. Preheat the oven to 400°F (200°C).

2. Arrange the fillets of salmon on a baking sheet.

3. Cover the salmon with a drizzle of lemon juice and olive oil.

4. Add a dash of pepper, salt, and dried dill.

5. 4. Bake the salmon for 15 to 20 minutes, or until it flake easily with a fork.

6. Present alongside some steaming broccoli.

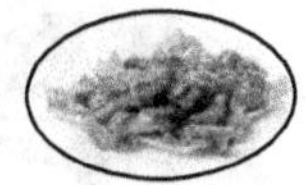 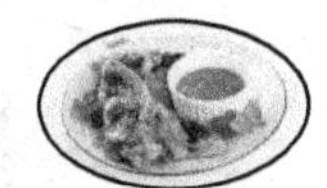 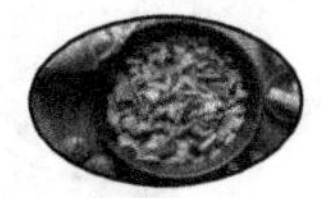

# Recipe 5: Turkey and Vegetable Stir-Fry

## Ingredients:

- 1 lb lean ground turkey
- 2 cups broccoli florets
- 1 bell pepper, sliced
- 1 carrot, julienned
- 2 tablespoons soy sauce
- 1 tablespoon sesame oil
- 1 teaspoon ginger, minced
- 2 cloves garlic, minced

## Instructions:

1. In a wok or large skillet, brown the ground turkey over medium heat.
2. Add broccoli, bell pepper, and carrot to the wok.

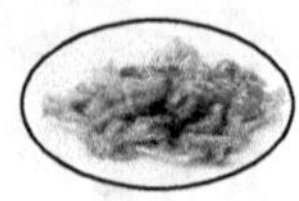 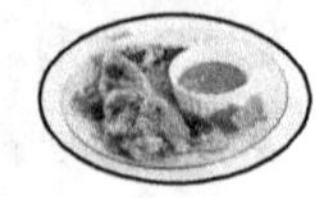 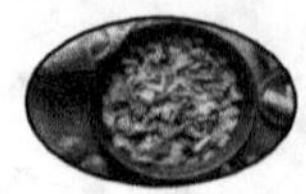

3.  In a small bowl, mix soy sauce, sesame oil, ginger, and garlic.

4.  Pour the sauce over the turkey and vegetables. Stir-fry until vegetables are tender.

5.  Serve over cauliflower rice.

## Recipe 6: Greek Yogurt Parfait

**Ingredients:**

- 2 cups Greek yogurt

- 1 cup mixed berries (strawberries, blueberries, raspberries)

- 1/4 cup granola

- 1 tablespoon honey

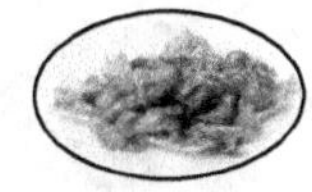 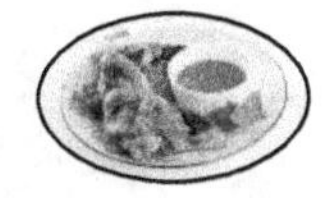 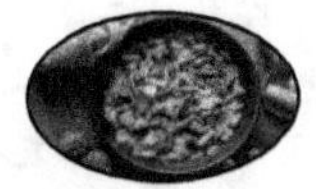

## Instructions:

1. . Arrange granola, mixed berries, and Greek yogurt in a glass or dish

2. Drizzle honey on top.

3. Repeat the layers.

4. Serve chilled.

## Recipe 7: Egg and Vegetable Breakfast Wrap

## Ingredients:

- 4 whole-grain tortillas

- 4 large eggs, scrambled

- 1 cup spinach, chopped

- 1 tomato, diced–

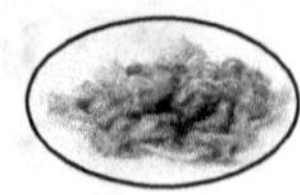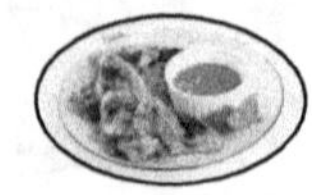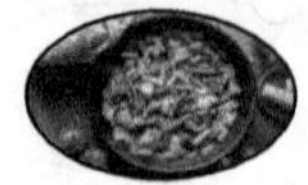

- 1/2 cup feta cheese, crumbled

- Salt and pepper to taste

## Instructions:

1. In a pan, scramble the eggs until cooked through.

2. Warm the tortillas in the same pan.

3. Divide the scrambled eggs among the tortillas.

4. Top with spinach, tomato, and feta cheese.

5. Season with salt and pepper.

6. Roll up the tortillas and serve.

## Recipe 8: Cauliflower Pizza Crust

### Ingredients:

- 1 head cauliflower, riced

- 1 cup mozzarella cheese, shredded–

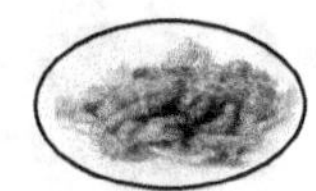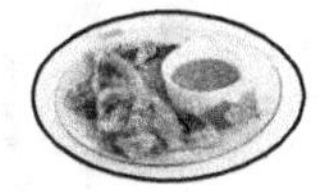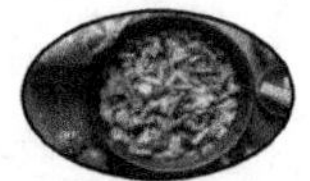

- 1 egg

- 1 teaspoon dried oregano

- 1/2 teaspoon garlic powder

- Tomato sauce, cheese, and toppings for pizza

**Instructions:**

1. Preheat the oven to 425°F (220°C).

2. Microwave or steam cauliflower until tender, then rice it using a food processor.

3. Mix cauliflower rice, mozzarella, egg, oregano, and garlic powder in a bowl.

4. Press the mixture onto a pizza stone or baking sheet to form a crust.

5. Bake for about twenty minutes or when a golden brown color is attained.

6. Add tomato sauce, cheese, and your favorite toppings.

7. Bake for an additional 10 minutes.

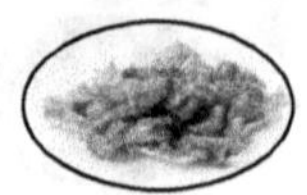 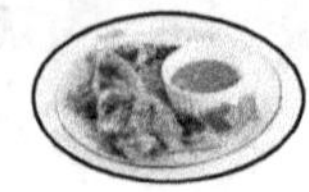 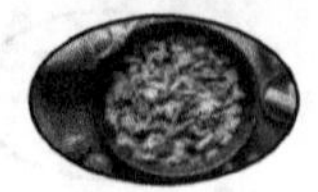



**Ingredients:**

- 4 bell peppers, halved

- 1 cup cooked quinoa

- 1 can black beans, drained and rinsed

- 1 cup corn kernels

- 1 cup salsa

- 1 teaspoon cumin

- 1/2 teaspoon chili powder

- 1 cup shredded cheddar cheese

—

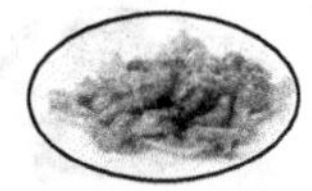 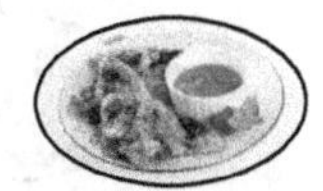 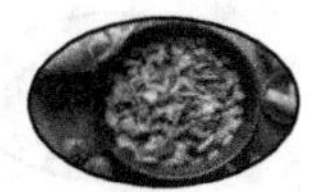

## Instructions:

1. Preheat the oven to 375°F (190°C).

2. In a bowl, mix quinoa, black beans, corn, salsa, cumin, and chili powder.

3. Stuff each pepper half with the quinoa mixture.

4. Top with shredded cheddar cheese.

5. Bake for 25-30 minutes or until the peppers are tender.

6. It should be Serve with a dollop of yogurt (Greek)

## Recipe 10: Lentil and Vegetable Soup

## Ingredients:

- 1 cup dried green lentils, rinsed

- 1 onion, chopped

- 2 carrots, diced–

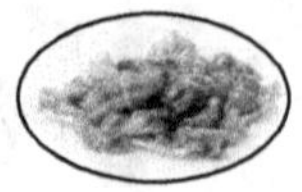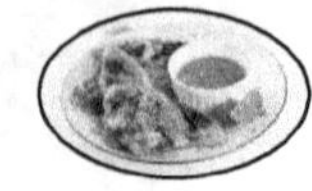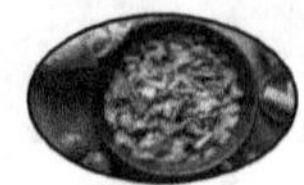

- 2 celery stalks, sliced

- 3 cloves garlic, minced

- 1 can diced tomatoes

- 6 cups vegetable broth

- 1 teaspoon cumin

- 1/2 teaspoon smoked paprika

- Salt and pepper to taste

## Instructions:

1. In a large pot, sauté onions, carrots, celery, and garlic until softened.

2. Add lentils, diced tomatoes, vegetable broth, cumin, smoked paprika, salt, and pepper.

3. Bring to a boil, then reduce heat and simmer for 25-30 minutes.

4. Adjust seasoning if needed.

5. Serve hot, optionally with a squeeze of fresh lemon juice.

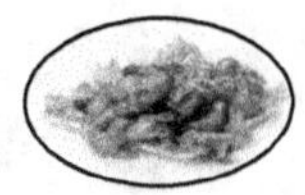 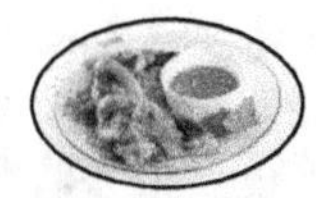 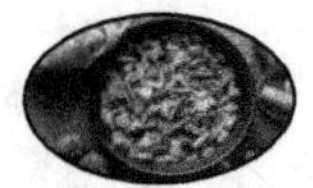

# Recipe 11: Shrimp and Asparagus Stir-Fry

**Ingredients:**

- 1 lb shrimp, peeled and deveined

- One bunch of asparagus, peeled and sliced into 2-inch segments

- 1 red bell pepper, sliced

- 2 tablespoons low-sodium soy sauce

- 1 tablespoon rice vinegar

- 1 tablespoon sesame oil

- 1 teaspoon honey

- 2 teaspoons cornstarch

- 2 cloves garlic, minced

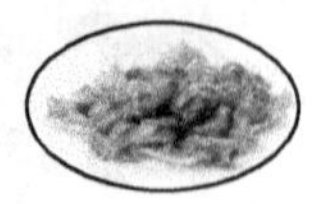 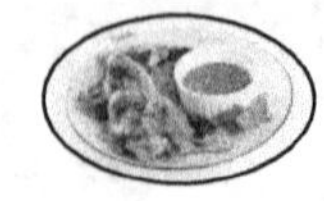 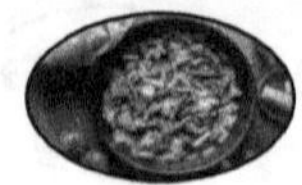

**Instructions:**

1. In a bowl, whisk together soy sauce, rice vinegar, sesame oil, honey, and cornstarch.

2. . Turn up the heat to medium-high in a large skillet.

3. Add shrimp and cook until pink, then remove from the pan.

4. In the same pan, stir-fry asparagus, bell pepper, and garlic until crisp-tender.

5. Return shrimp to the pan and pour the sauce over the mixture.

6. Toss everything until well coated and heated through.

7. Serve over brown rice.

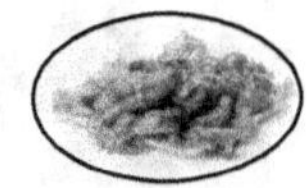 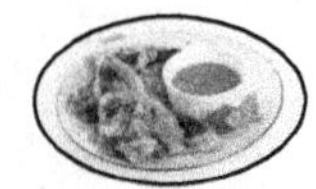 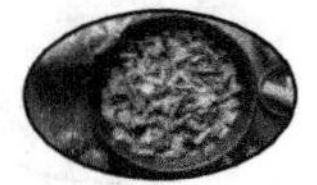

# Recipe 12: Sweet Potato and Chickpea

## Buddha Bowl

**Ingredients:**

- 2 sweet potatoes, diced

- 1 can chickpeas, drained and rinsed

- 2 cups kale, chopped

- 1 avocado, sliced

- 1/4 cup tahini

- Juice of 1 lemon

- 2 tablespoons olive oil

- Salt and pepper to taste

**Instructions:**

1. Preheat the oven to 400°F (200°C).

2. Toss sweet potatoes and chickpeas with olive oil, salt, and pepper.

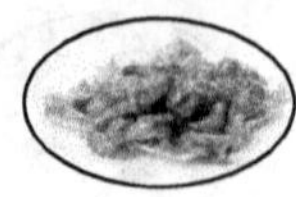 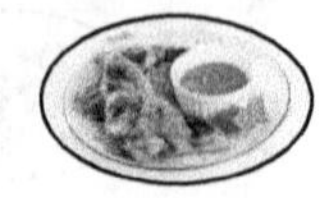 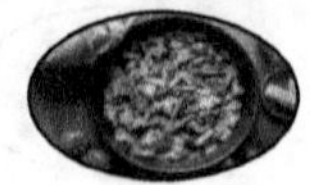

3. Bake/roast for 25 to 30 minutes, or until brown.

4. In a bowl, massage kale with lemon juice.

5. Assemble bowls with roasted sweet potatoes, chickpeas, kale, and sliced avocado.

6. Drizzle with tahini.

7. Enjoy!

## Recipe 13: Chicken and Vegetable Skewers

**Ingredients:**

- cut into cubes ,1 lb. chicken breast

- 1 zucchini, sliced

- 1 red onion, cut into chunks

- 1 bell pepper, cut into squares

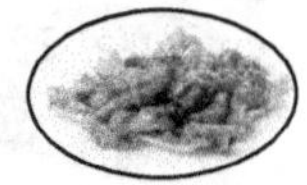 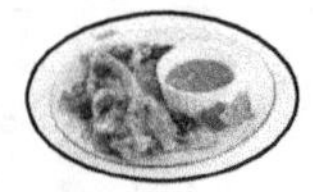 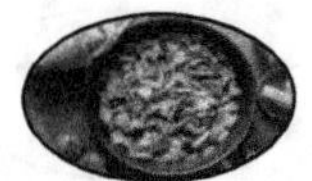

- 2 tablespoons olive oil

- 1 teaspoon Italian seasoning

- Salt and pepper to taste

**Instructions:**

1. Preheat the grill or grill pan.

2. Thread chicken, zucchini, red onion, and bell pepper onto skewers.

3. In a small bowl, mix olive oil, Italian seasoning, salt, and pepper.

4. Brush the skewers with the oil mixture.

5. Grill for 10-12 minutes, turning occasionally, until the chicken is cooked through.

6. . Accompany with quinoa or brown rice on the side.

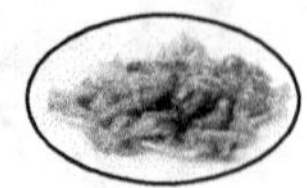 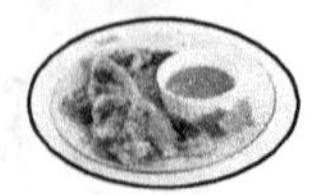 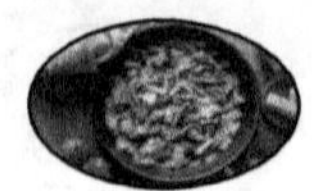

# Recipe 14: Caprese Stuffed Chicken Breast

**Ingredients:**

- 4 chicken breasts

- 1 cup cherry tomatoes, halved

- 4 oz fresh mozzarella, sliced

- 1/4 cup fresh basil leaves

- 2 tablespoons balsamic glaze

- Salt and pepper to taste

**Instructions:**

1. Preheat the oven to 375°F (190°C).

2. Slit each chicken breast into a pocket.

3. Stuff mozzarella, basil, and tomatoes into each pocket.

4. Add salt and pepper to the chicken's seasoning.

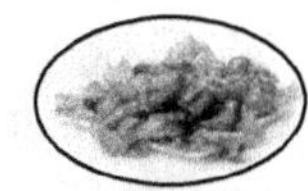 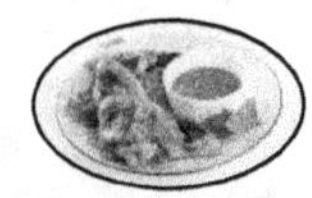 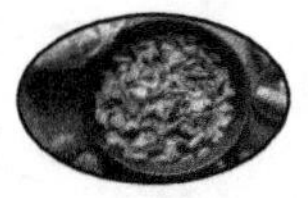

5. Transfer the filled chicken breasts to an ovenproof tray.

6. Bake for 25-30 minutes or until the chicken is cooked through.

7. Drizzle with balsamic glaze before serving.

## Recipe 15: Broccoli and Cheddar Stuffed Potatoes

**Ingredients:**

- 4 medium-sized potatoes, baked

- 2 cups broccoli florets, steamed

- 1 cup shredded cheddar cheese

- 1/2 cup Greek yogurt

- Salt and pepper to taste–

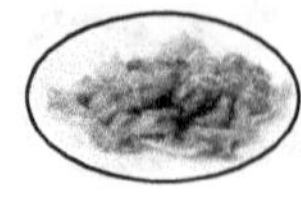 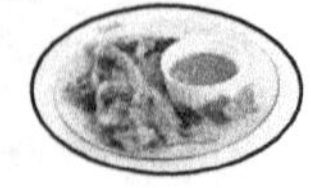 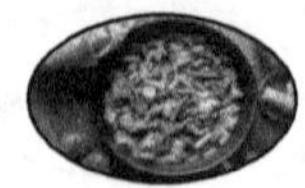

**Instructions:**

1. Cut a slit in each baked potato and fluff the insides with a fork.

2. In a bowl, mix steamed broccoli, cheddar cheese,Greek yogurt, salt, and pepper.

3. Stuff each potato with the broccoli and cheddar mixture.

4. Place the stuffed potatoes back in the oven for 5 minutes to melt the cheese.

5. Serve hot.–

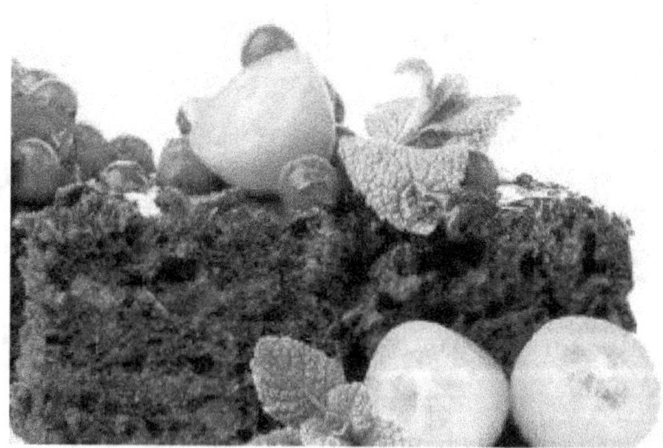

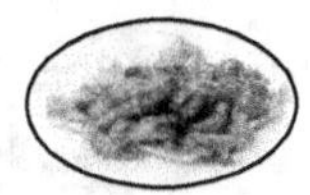 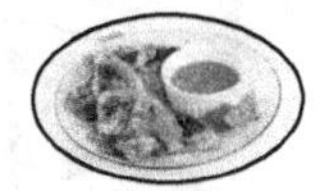 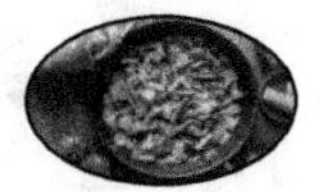

# Recipe 16: Turkey and Quinoa Stuffed Acorn Squash

**Ingredients:**

- 2 acorn squash, halved and seeds removed
- 1 cup cooked quinoa
- 1 lb ground turkey
- 1 onion, diced
- 2 cloves garlic, minced
- 1 teaspoon dried sage
- 1/2 teaspoon cinnamon
- Salt and pepper to taste

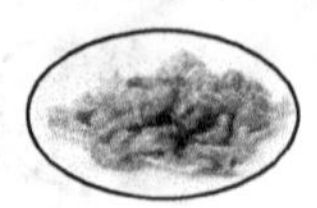 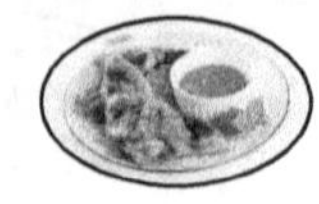 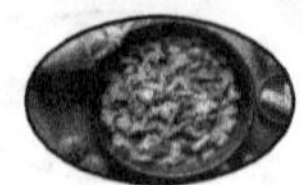

**Instructions:**

1. Preheat the oven to 375°F (190°C).

2. Place acorn squash halves on a baking sheet, cut side down.

3. Bake for 25-30 minutes or until tender.

4. In a pan, cook ground turkey, onion, and garlic until turkey is browned.

5. Stir in cooked quinoa, sage, cinnamon, salt, and pepper.

6. Stuff each acorn squash half with the turkey and quinoa mixture.

7. Bake for an additional 15 minutes.

8. Enjoy your hearty stuffed squash!

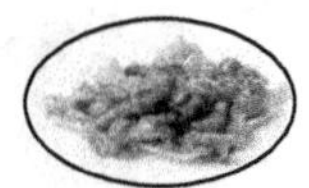 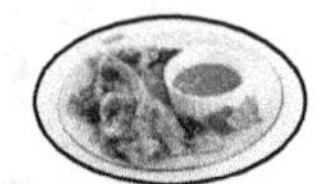 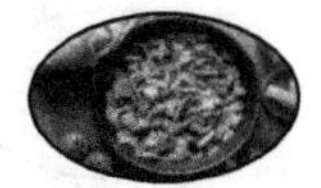

# Recipe 17: Spinach and Mushroom Omelette

**Ingredients:**

- 4 eggs
- 1 cup spinach, chopped
- 1/2 cup mushrooms, sliced
- 1/4 cup feta cheese, crumbled
- 1 tablespoon olive oil
- Salt and pepper to taste

**Instructions:**

1. Combine eggs, salt, and pepper in a bowl.
2. In a nonstick skillet, warm the olive oil over medium heat.
3. Sauté mushrooms until golden, then add spinach and cook until wilted.

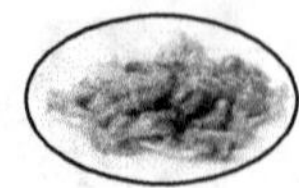 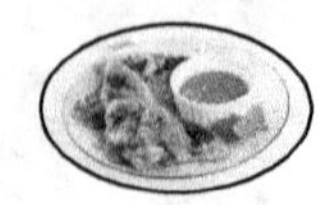 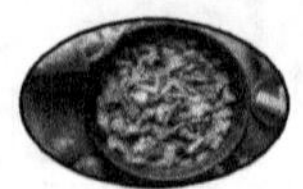

4. Pour the whisked eggs over the vegetables.

5. Sprinkle feta cheese on top.

6. Cook until the edges set, then fold the omelette in half.

7. Slide onto a plate and serve.

## Recipe 18: Berry and Almond Smoothie Bowl

**Ingredients:**

- 1 cup mixed berries (strawberries, blueberries, raspberries)

- 1 banana, sliced

- 1/4 cup almond butter

- 1 cup unsweetened almond milk

- 1 tablespoon chia seeds

- Granola for topping

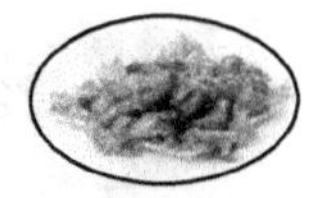 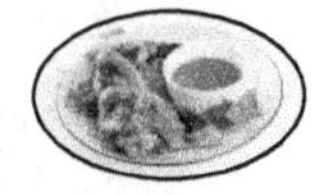 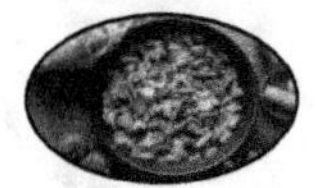

## Instructions:

1. In a blender, combine mixed berries, banana, almond butter, and almond milk.

2. Blend until smooth.

3. Pour the smoothie into a bowl.

4. Top with chia seeds and granola.

5. Enjoy a nutritious and delicious smoothie bowl!

## Recipe 19: Cabbage and Chicken Stir-Fry

## Ingredients:

- 1 lb chicken thighs, thinly sliced

- 1 small cabbage, shredded

- 2 carrots, julienned

- 1 bell pepper, sliced

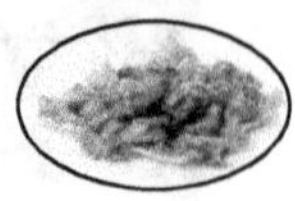 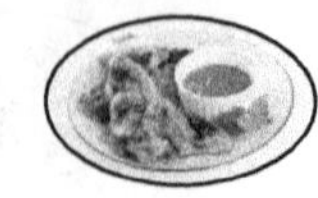 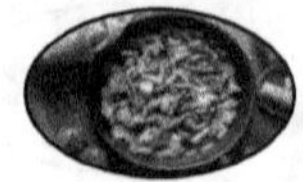

- 2 tablespoons soy sauce

- 1 tablespoon hoisin sauce

- 1 tablespoon sesame oil

- 1 teaspoon ginger, minced

- 2 cloves garlic, minced

## Instructions:

1. In a wok or large skillet, cook sliced chicken until browned.

2. Add cabbage, carrots, and bell pepper to the wok.

3. In a small bowl, mix soy sauce, hoisin sauce, sesame oil, ginger, and garlic.

4. Combine eggs, salt, and pepper in a bowl.

5. In a nonstick skillet, warm the olive oil over medium heat.

6. Stir-fry until the vegetables are tender.

7. Serve over brown rice or cauliflower rice.–

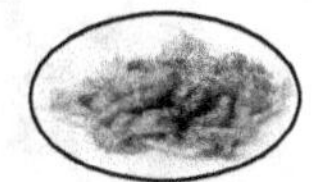 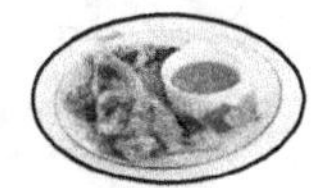 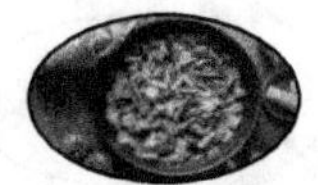

# Recipe 20: Avocado and Black Bean Salad

## Ingredients:

- 2 avocados, diced

- 1 can black beans, drained and rinsed

- 1 cup corn kernels

- 1 cup cherry tomatoes, halved

- 1/4 cup red onion, finely chopped

- 2 tablespoons lime juice

- 2 tablespoons cilantro, chopped

- Salt and pepper to taste

## Instructions:

1. In a large bowl, combine diced avocados, black beans, corn, cherry tomatoes, and red onion.

2. Drizzle lime juice over the mixture.

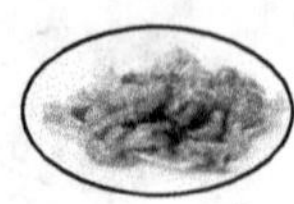 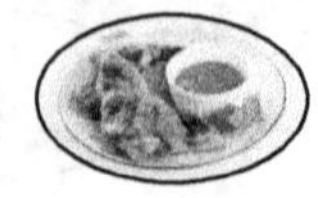 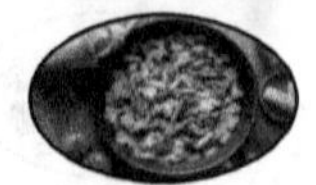

3.  Add chopped cilantro, salt, and pepper.

4.  Toss gently to combine.

5.  Serve as a refreshing salad or as a side dish.

# Recipe 21: Turkey and Sweet Potato Chili

**Ingredients:**

- 1 lb ground turkey

- 2 sweet potatoes, peeled and diced

- 1 can black beans, drained and rinsed

- 1 can diced tomatoes

- 1 onion, chopped

- 2 cloves garlic, minced

- 1 tablespoon chili powder

- 1 teaspoon cumin

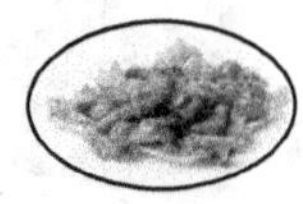 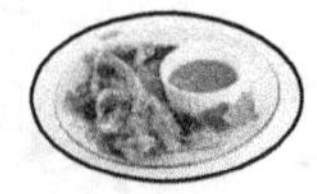 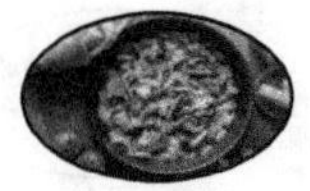

- Salt and pepper to taste

- Greek yogurt, grated cheese, and chopped green onions are optional garnishes.

## Instructions:

1. In a large pot, brown ground turkey over medium heat.

2. Add onions and garlic, sauté until softened.

3. Stir in sweet potatoes, black beans, diced tomatoes, chili powder, cumin, salt, and pepper.

4. Simmer for 20-25 minutes or until sweet potatoes are tender.

5. Adjust seasoning if needed.

6. Serve hot with your favorite toppings.

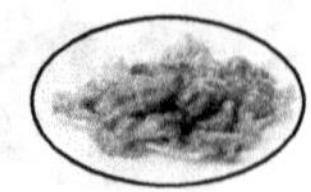 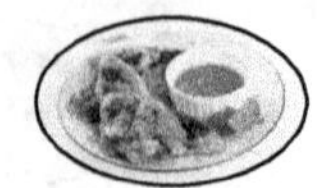 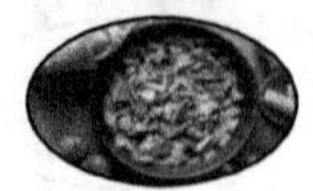



**Ingredients:**

- One block of diced and pressed firm tofu

- 2 cups broccoli florets

- 1 bell pepper, sliced

- 1 carrot, julienned

- 2 tablespoons soy sauce

- 1 tablespoon hoisin sauce

- 1 tablespoon sesame oil

- 1 teaspoon ginger, minced

- 2 cloves garlic, minced

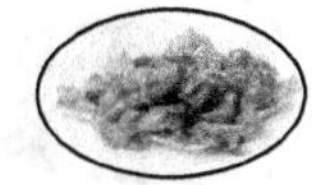 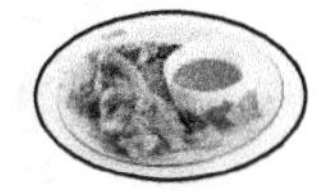 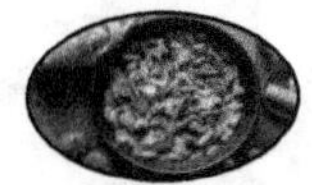

**Instructions:**

1. In a wok or large skillet, sauté cubed tofu until golden.

2. Add broccoli, bell pepper, and carrot to the wok.

3. In a small bowl, mix soy sauce, hoisin sauce, sesame oil, ginger, and garlic.

4. Pour the sauce over the tofu and vegetables.

5. Stir-fry until vegetables are tender and tofu is coated.

6. Serve over brown rice or quinoa.

## Recipe 23: Pesto and Chicken Zoodle Bowl

**Ingredients:**

- 2 zucchinis, spiralized

- 1 lb chicken breast, cooked and sliced

- 1 cup cherry tomatoes, halved

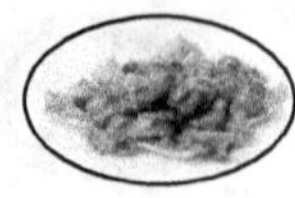 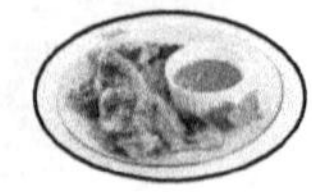 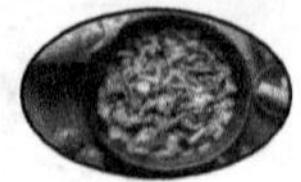

- 1/4 cup pesto sauce

- 2 tablespoons pine nuts

- Salt and pepper to taste

- Optional: grated Parmesan cheese

## Instructions:

1. In a pan, sauté spiralized zucchini until tender.

2. Add cooked chicken and cherry tomatoes to the pan.

3. Stir in pesto sauce and cook until everything is heated through.

4. Season with salt and pepper.

5. Top with pine nuts and, if desired, grated Parmesan.

6. Serve warm.–

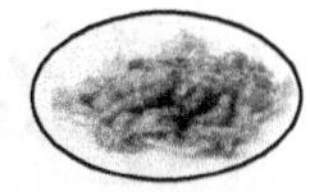 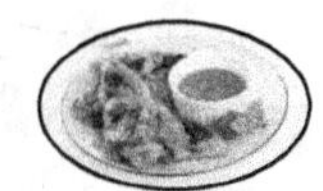 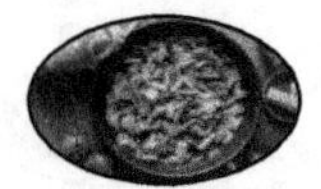

# Recipe 24: Spaghetti Squash with Marinara Sauce

**Ingredients:**

- One spaghetti squash, cut in half, and seeded

- 2 cups marinara sauce

- 1 tablespoon olive oil

- 1 teaspoon dried Italian herbs

- Salt and pepper to taste

- Fresh basil for garnish

**Instructions:**

1. Preheat the oven to 400°F (200°C).

2. Brush the cut sides of the spaghetti squash with olive oil.

3. . Add some salt, pepper, and dry herbs.

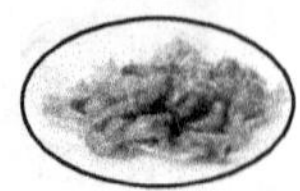 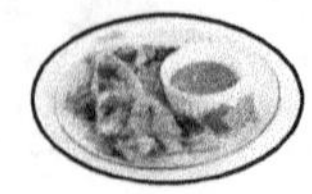 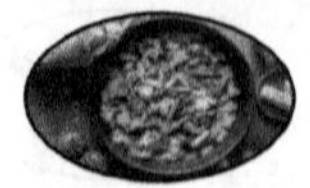

4. Roast in the oven for 40-45 minutes or until the squash is fork-tender.

5. Scrape the flesh with a fork to create "spaghetti."

6. Heat marinara sauce and pour it over the spaghetti squash.

7. Garnish with fresh basil and serve.

## Recipe 25: Blueberry and Almond Overnight Oats

**Ingredients:**

- 1/2 cup rolled oats

- 1/2 cup almond milk

- 1/4 cup Greek yogurt

- 1/4 cup fresh blueberries

- 1 tablespoon almond butter

- 1 teaspoon chia seeds

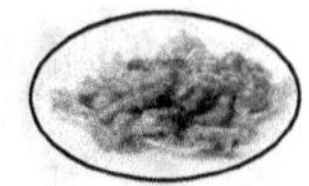 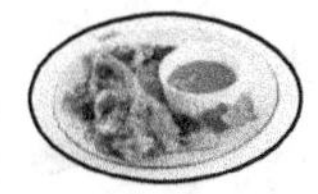 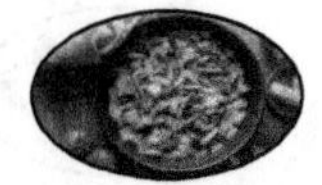

- 1 teaspoon honey

## Instructions:

1. In a jar, combine rolled oats, almond milk, Greek yogurt, chia seeds, and honey.

2. Stir well and refrigerate overnight.

3. In the morning, top with fresh blueberries and a dollop of almond butter.

4. Mix before enjoying your delicious and nutritious breakfast.

## Recipe 26: Eggplant and Tomato Casserole

## Ingredients:

- 2 eggplants, sliced

- 2 cups cherry tomatoes, halved–

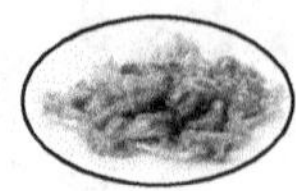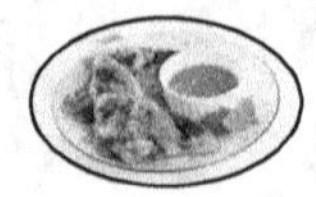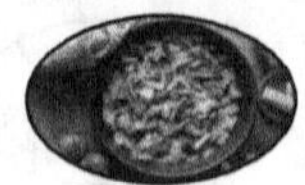

- 1 cup mozzarella cheese, shredded

- 1/4 cup fresh basil, chopped

- 2 tablespoons olive oil

- 2 cloves garlic, minced

- Salt and pepper to taste

**Instructions:**

1. Preheat the oven to 375°F (190°C).

2. Brush eggplant slices with olive oil and arrange them in a baking dish.

3. In a bowl, mix cherry tomatoes, mozzarella, basil, garlic, salt, and pepper.

4. Spread the tomato mixture over the eggplant.

5. Bake for 25-30 minutes or until the cheese is bubbly and golden.

6. Serve as a flavorful side dish.–

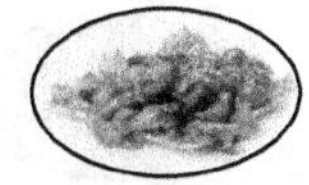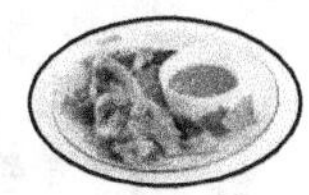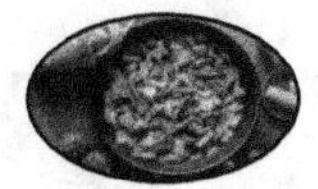

# Recipe 27: Quinoa and Black Bean Stuffed Bell Peppers

**Ingredients:**

- 4 bell peppers, halved

- 1 cup cooked quinoa

- 1 can black beans, drained and rinsed

- 1 cup corn kernels

- 1 cup salsa

- 1 teaspoon cumin

- 1/2 teaspoon chili powder

- 1 cup shredded Monterey Jack cheese

**Instructions:**

1. Preheat the oven to 375°F (190°C).

2. In a bowl, mix quinoa, black beans, corn, salsa, cumin, and chili powder.

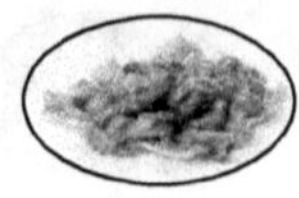 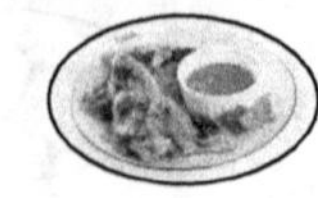 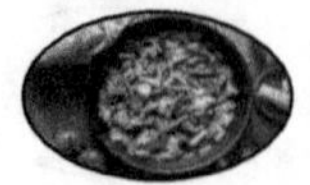

3. Stuff each bell pepper half with the quinoa mixture.

4. Top with shredded Monterey Jack cheese.

5. Bake for 25-30 minutes or until the peppers are tender.

6. . Accompany with a mound of Greek yogurt.

## Recipe 28: Turkey and Veggie Lettuce Wraps

**Ingredients:**

- 1 lb ground turkey

- 1 bell pepper, finely diced

- 1 zucchini, grated

- 2 tablespoons soy sauce

- 1 tablespoon hoisin sauce–

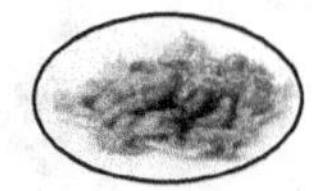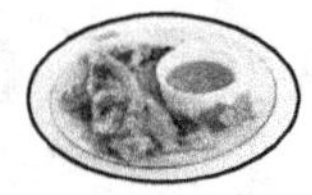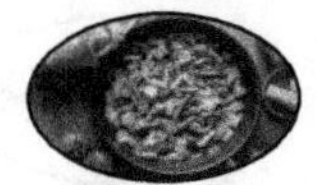

- 1 teaspoon sesame oil

- 1 teaspoon ginger, minced

- 1 clove garlic, minced

- Leaves of iceberg or butter lettuce, for wrapping

**Instructions:**

1. In a pan, brown ground turkey over medium heat.

2. Add bell pepper and zucchini, sauté until softened.

3. In a small bowl, mix soy sauce, hoisin sauce, sesame oil, ginger, and garlic.

4. Pour the sauce over the turkey and vegetables, stir well.

5. Spoon the turkey mixture into lettuce leaves to create wraps.

6. Enjoy a flavorful and low-carb meal.–

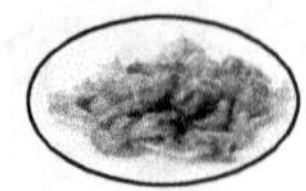 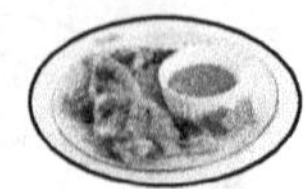 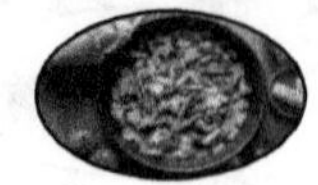



## Ingredients:

- 2 cans chickpeas, drained and rinsed

- 1 cucumber, diced

- 1 cup cherry tomatoes, halved

- 1/2 red onion, finely chopped

- 1/4 cup Kalamata olives, sliced

- 1/4 cup feta cheese, crumbled

- 2 tablespoons olive oil

- 1 tablespoon red wine vinegar

- 1 teaspoon dried oregano

- Salt and pepper to taste–

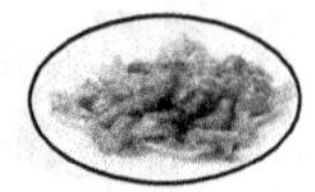 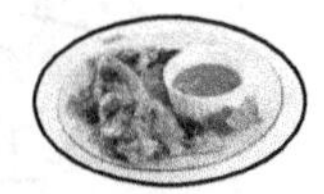 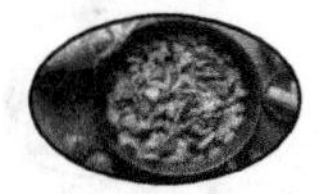

## Instructions:

1. In a large bowl, combine chickpeas, cucumber, cherry tomatoes, red onion, olives, and feta cheese.

2. Combine the olive oil, red wine vinegar, oregano, salt, and pepper in a small bowl.

3. Drizzle the salad with the dressing and gently mix.

4. Let it cool for a minimum of half an hour before serving.

5. Serve as a refreshing and protein-packed salad.

## Recipe 30: Butternut Squash and Sage Risotto

## Ingredients:

- 1 cup Arborio rice

- 3 cups butternut squash, diced–

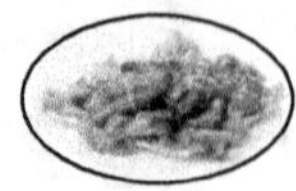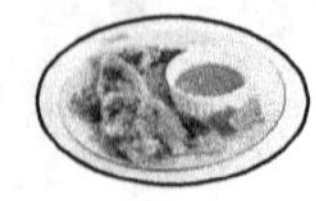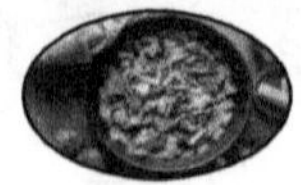

- 1 onion, finely chopped

- 2 cloves garlic, minced

- 1/2 cup dry white wine

- 4 cups vegetable broth, heated

- 2 tablespoons olive oil

- 1 tablespoon fresh sage, chopped

- Salt and pepper to taste

- Grated Parmesan cheese for topping

**Instructions:**

1. In a large pan, sauté onion and garlic in olive oil until translucent.

2. Add Arborio rice and stir for 1-2 minutes.

3. Pour in white wine and let it cook until mostly absorbed.

4. Begin adding warm vegetable broth one ladle at a time, stirring frequently.

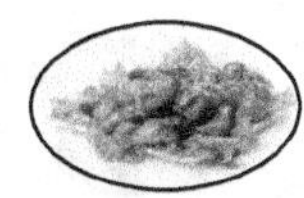 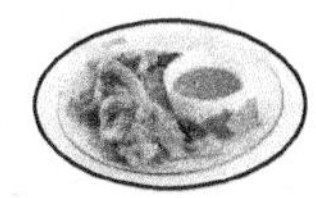 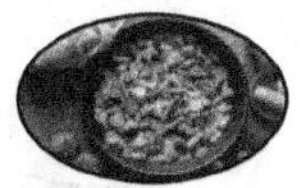

5. Add diced butternut squash and continue adding broth until the rice is creamy and cooked to al dente.

6. Stir in chopped sage, salt, and pepper.

7. Top with grated Parmesan cheese before serving.

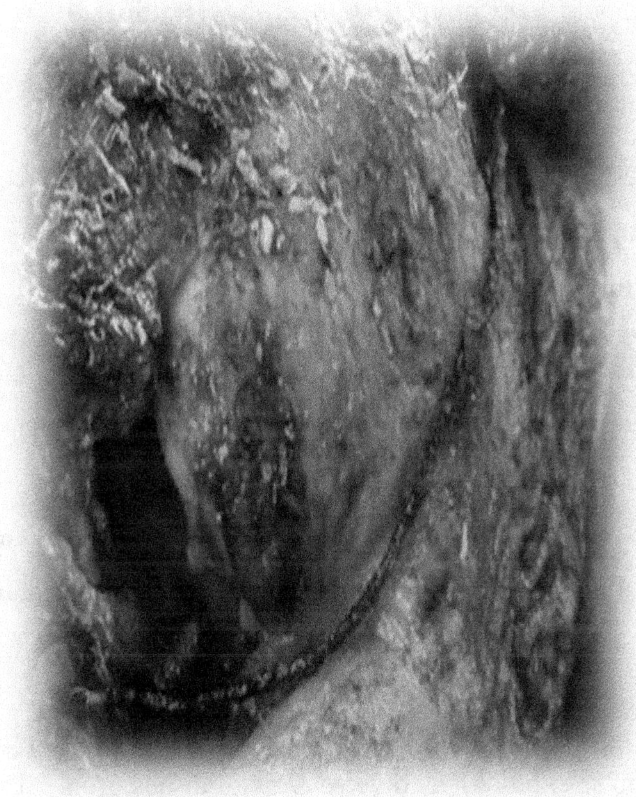

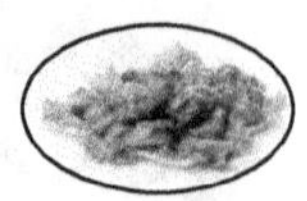 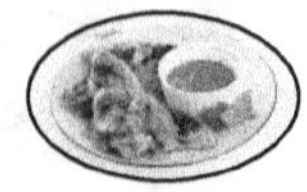 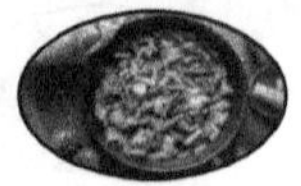

# CONCLUSION

**Nourishing Your Future**

As we reach the final pages of the "Type 1 Diabetes Cookbook: A Complete Guide for Healthy Living by Balancing Your Blood Sugar," it is our sincere hope that this culinary journey has been more than just a collection of recipes. We aspire for it to be a companion, a source of inspiration, and a testament to the transformative power of mindful eating.

In these pages, you've discovered that managing Type 1 diabetes isn't just about restriction; it's about embracing a world of flavors, textures, and nourishment that aligns with your health goals. Each recipe has been crafted with precision, keeping in mind the delicate balance needed to maintain stable blood sugar levels without compromising on taste or satisfaction.

As you've explored the diverse array of dishes, from vibrant salads to comforting casseroles, we trust that you've experienced the joy of a well-balanced meal. More than just

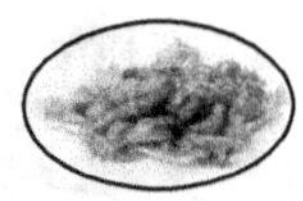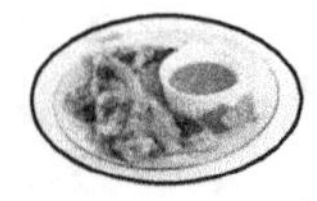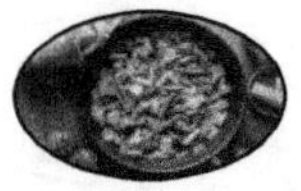

sustenance, these recipes are a celebration of life, a reminder that you have the power to nourish your body and soul with every mindful bite.

Remember, this cookbook is not a conclusion but a starting point—an invitation to continue exploring the limitless possibilities of a diabetes-friendly culinary landscape. We encourage you to experiment, personalize, and make these recipes your own. Whether you are newly diagnosed or a seasoned warrior in the fight against Type 1 diabetes, let this book be a guide on your path to wellness.

In closing, we extend our heartfelt gratitude for allowing us to be a part of your journey. May these recipes be a constant source of inspiration, empowerment, and joy in your pursuit of a healthy and fulfilling life. Here's to nourishing your future—one delicious and balanced meal at a time.

Wishing you good health, happiness, and flavorful adventures ahead.

Bon appétit and be well!

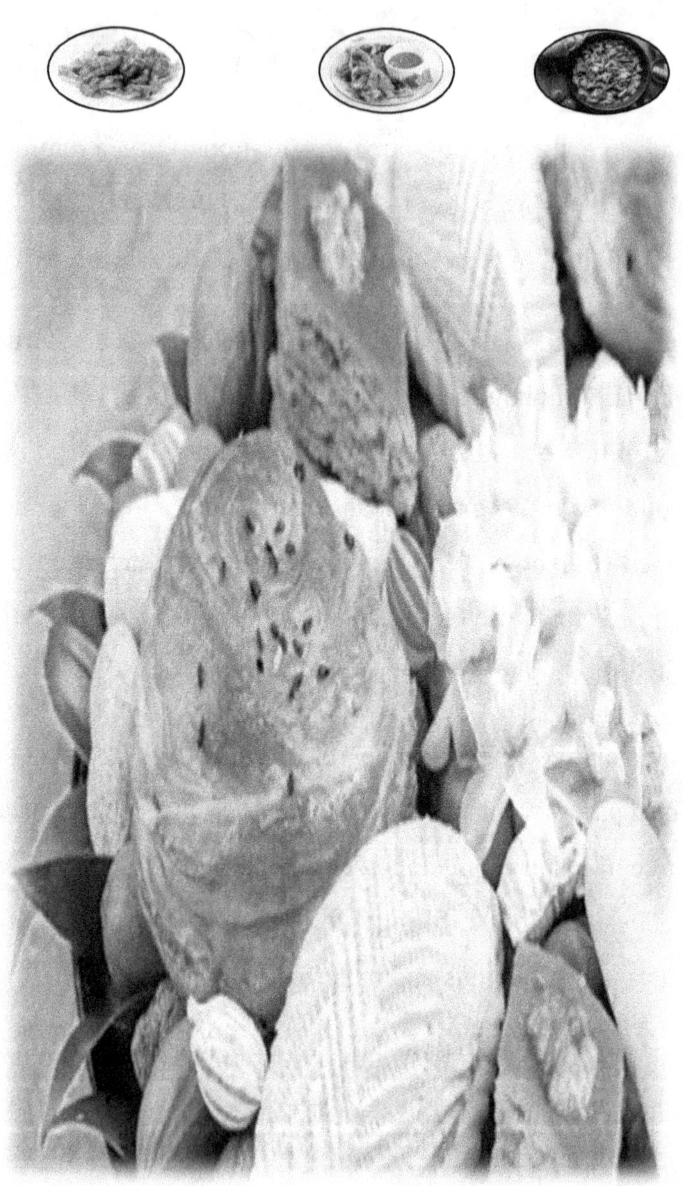

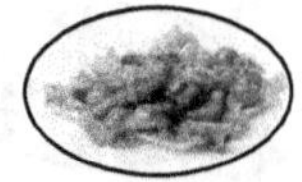 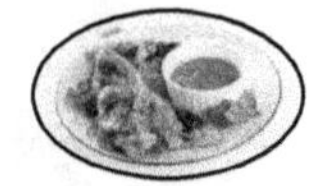 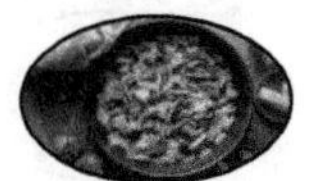

## WE KNOW...

*THAT'S WHY WE ARE SAYING THANK YOU...*

*"We know time is the unit of destiny, that's why we are saying thank you."*

*Dear Valued Customer,*

*we understand that time is a precious commodity, and we sincerely appreciate you choosing to spend a portion of it with us. Your decision to trust us with your purchase means the world to us, and we want to express our deepest gratitude.*

*Your support not only fuels our passion for delivering quality products but also contributes to the destiny of our business. Each customer is a vital part of our journey, and we are honored to have you*

*We strive to provide an exceptional shopping experience, and your satisfaction is our top priority. If you have any feedback or suggestions, we would love to hear from you. Your insights help us improve.*

*As a small token of our appreciation, we kindly invite you to share your experience by leaving a 5-star review. Your feedback not only boosts our morale but also assists fellow shoppers in making informed decisions.*

*Once again, thank you for choosing to buy this book. We look forward to serving you again and being a part of your destiny in the world of quality and excellence.*

*Warm regards,*

*Dr. Grace Hester–*

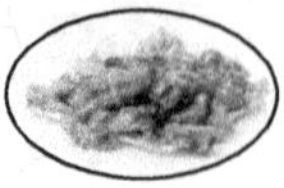

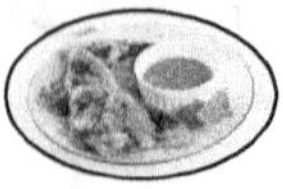

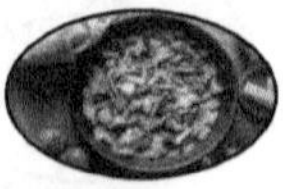

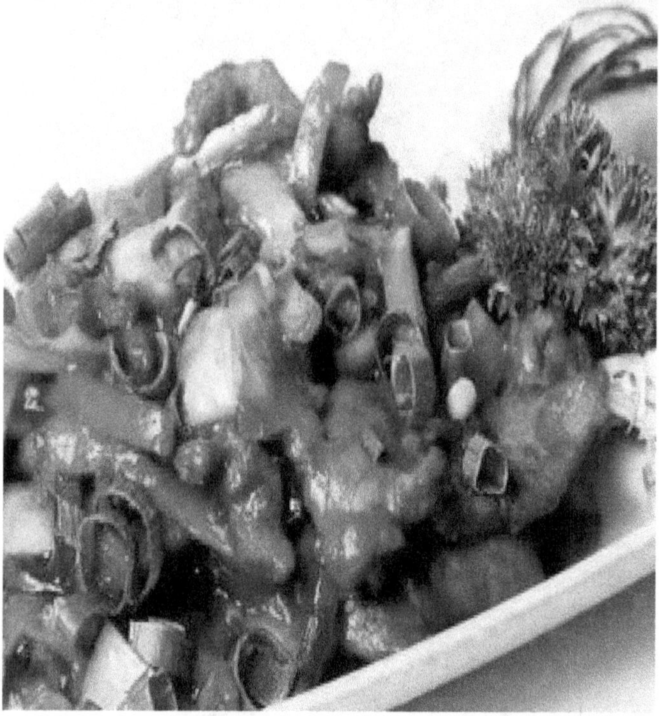

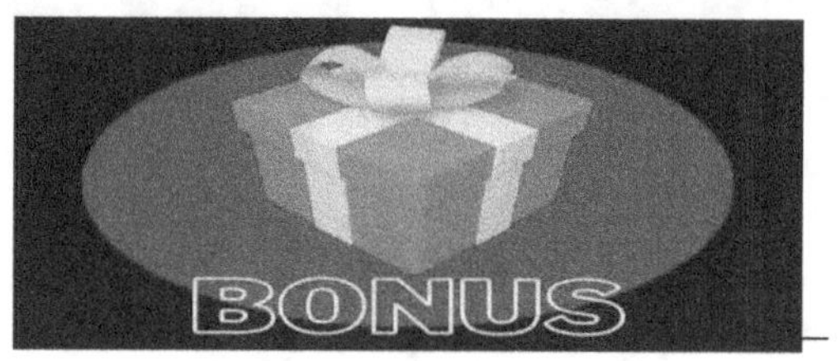

BONUS

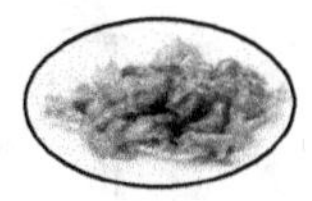 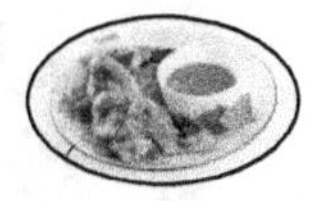 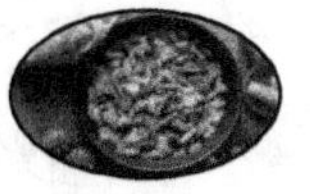

# BONUS 2; MICROWAVE COOKBOOK FOR DIABETIC PATIENTS

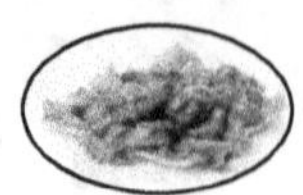 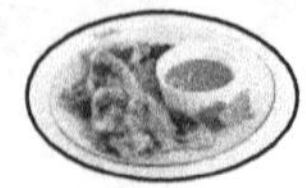 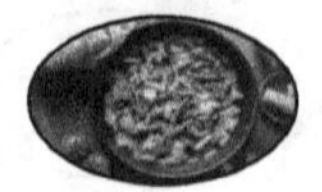

SCAN ME

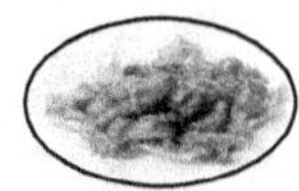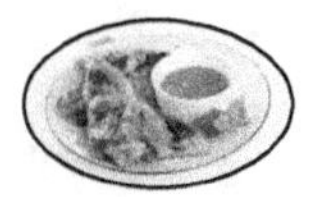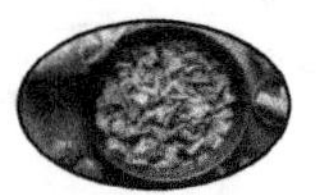

# BONUS 4;

# 20 DAYS + MEAL PLANNER

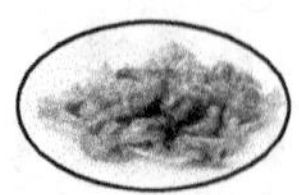 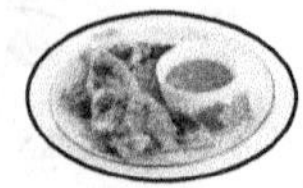 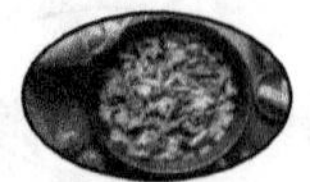

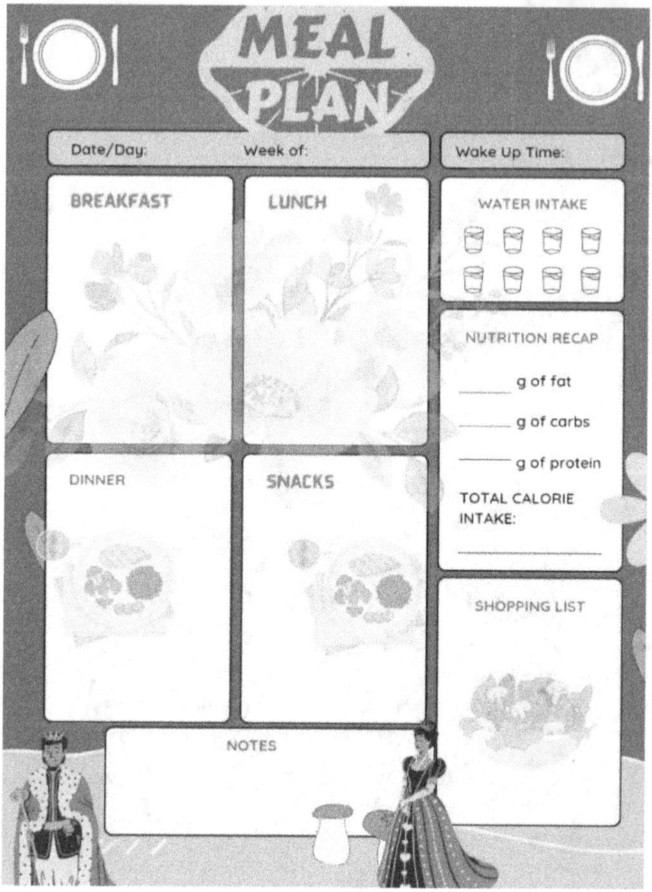

# MEAL PLAN

| Date/Day: | Week of: | Wake Up Time: |

## BREAKFAST

## LUNCH

### WATER INTAKE

### NUTRITION RECAP

__________ g of fat

__________ g of carbs

__________ g of protein

TOTAL CALORIE INTAKE:

__________

## DINNER

## SNACKS

### SHOPPING LIST

### NOTES

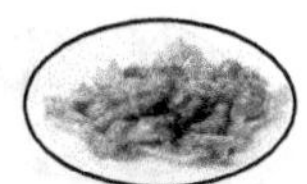 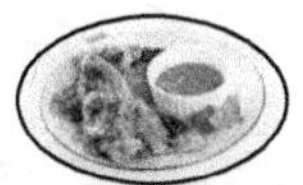 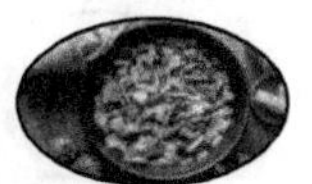

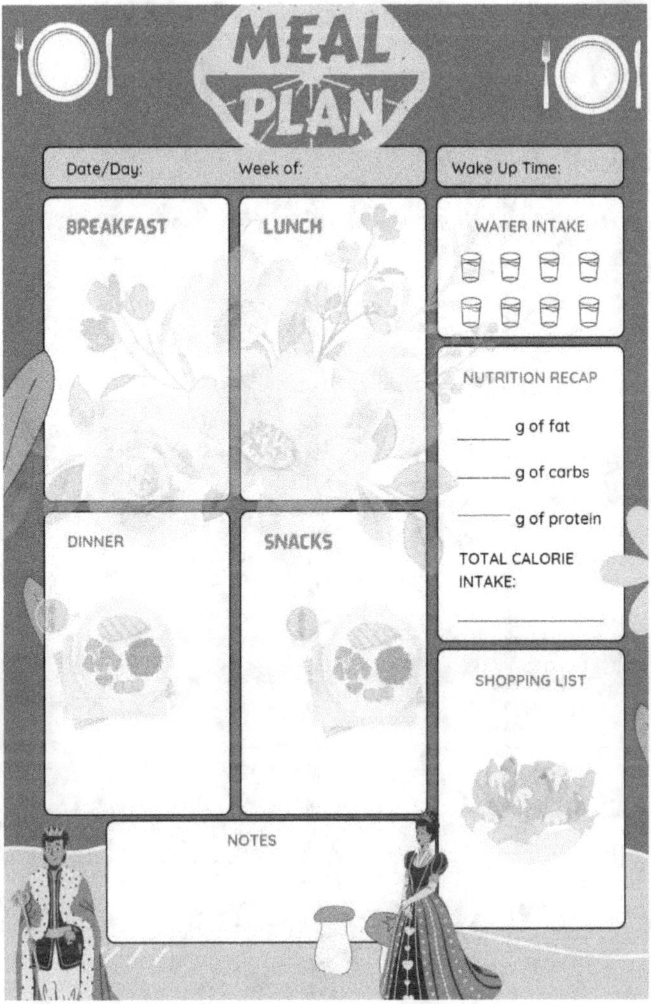

# MEAL PLAN

| Date/Day: | Week of: | Wake Up Time: |

## BREAKFAST

## LUNCH

## WATER INTAKE

## NUTRITION RECAP

_______ g of fat

_______ g of carbs

_______ g of protein

TOTAL CALORIE INTAKE:

_______________

## DINNER

## SNACKS

## SHOPPING LIST

## NOTES

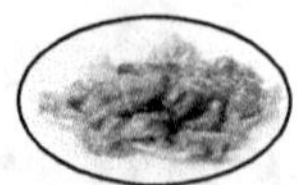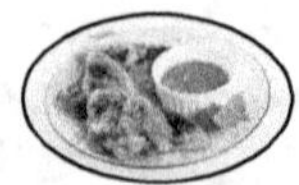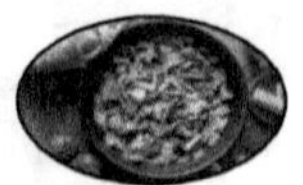

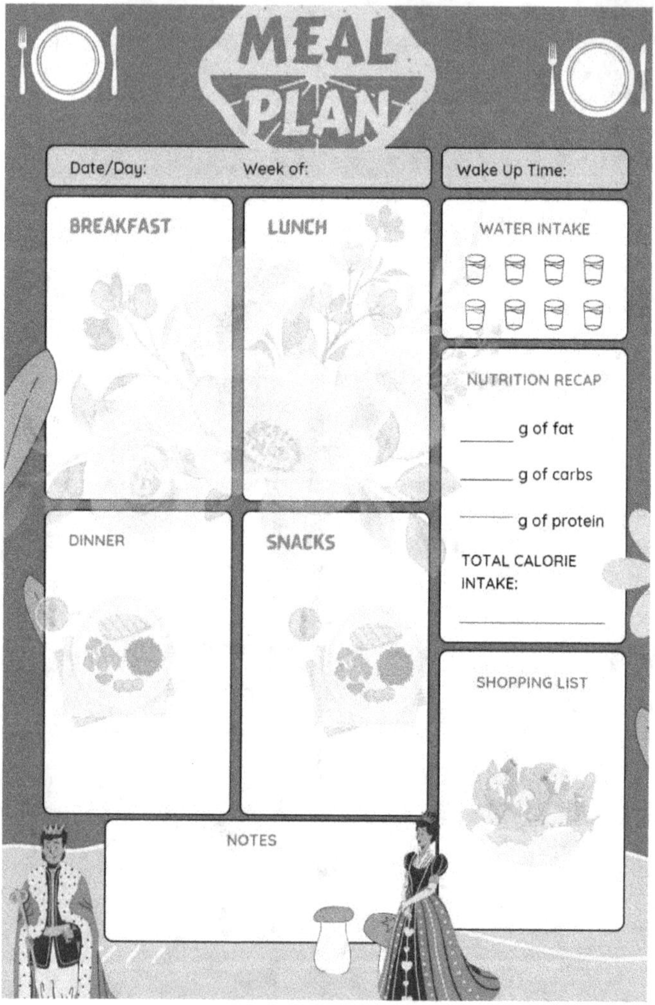

# MEAL PLAN

| Date/Day: | Week of: | Wake Up Time: |

## BREAKFAST

## LUNCH

### WATER INTAKE

### NUTRITION RECAP

_______ g of fat

_______ g of carbs

_______ g of protein

TOTAL CALORIE INTAKE:

_______________

## DINNER

## SNACKS

### SHOPPING LIST

### NOTES

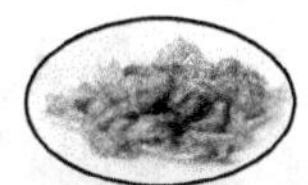 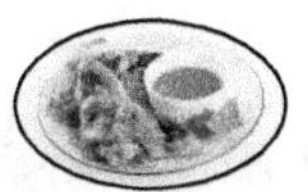 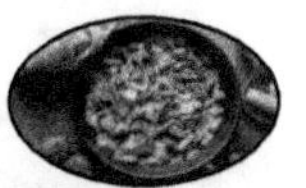

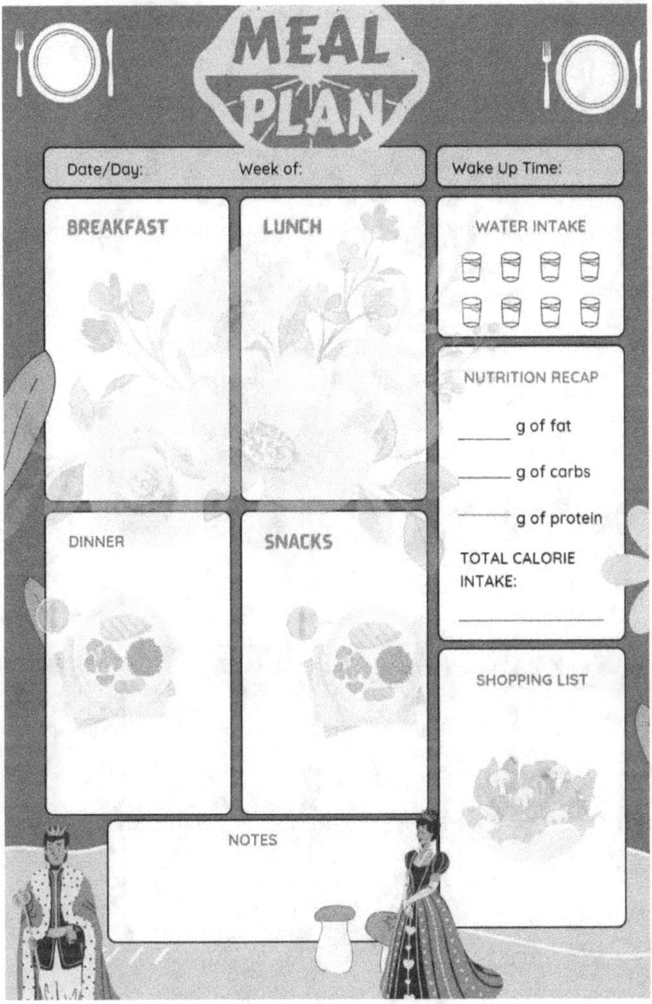

# MEAL PLAN

| Date/Day: | Week of: | Wake Up Time: |

## BREAKFAST

## LUNCH

### WATER INTAKE

### NUTRITION RECAP

_______ g of fat

_______ g of carbs

_______ g of protein

TOTAL CALORIE INTAKE:

_______________

## DINNER

## SNACKS

### SHOPPING LIST

### NOTES

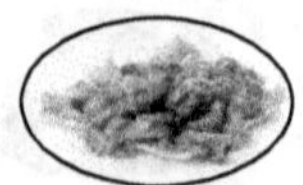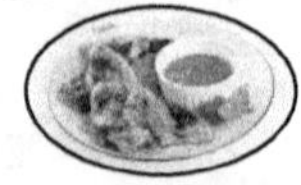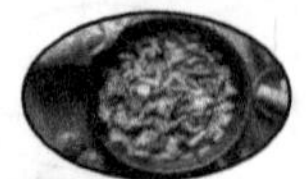

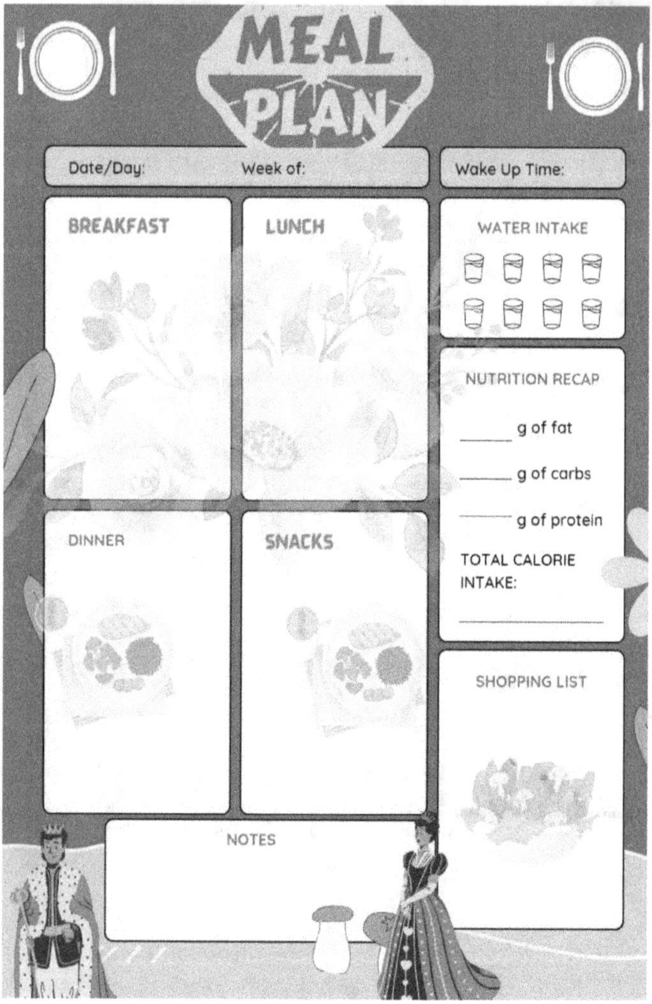

# MEAL PLAN

| Date/Day: | Week of: | Wake Up Time: |

### BREAKFAST

### LUNCH

### WATER INTAKE

### NUTRITION RECAP

______ g of fat

______ g of carbs

______ g of protein

TOTAL CALORIE INTAKE:

______

### DINNER

### SNACKS

### SHOPPING LIST

### NOTES

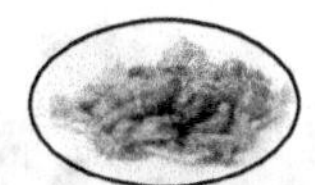 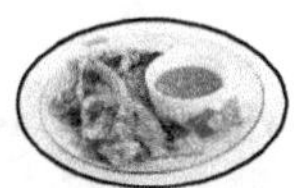 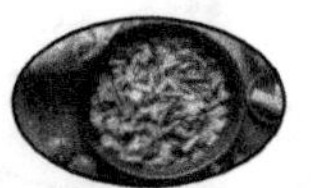

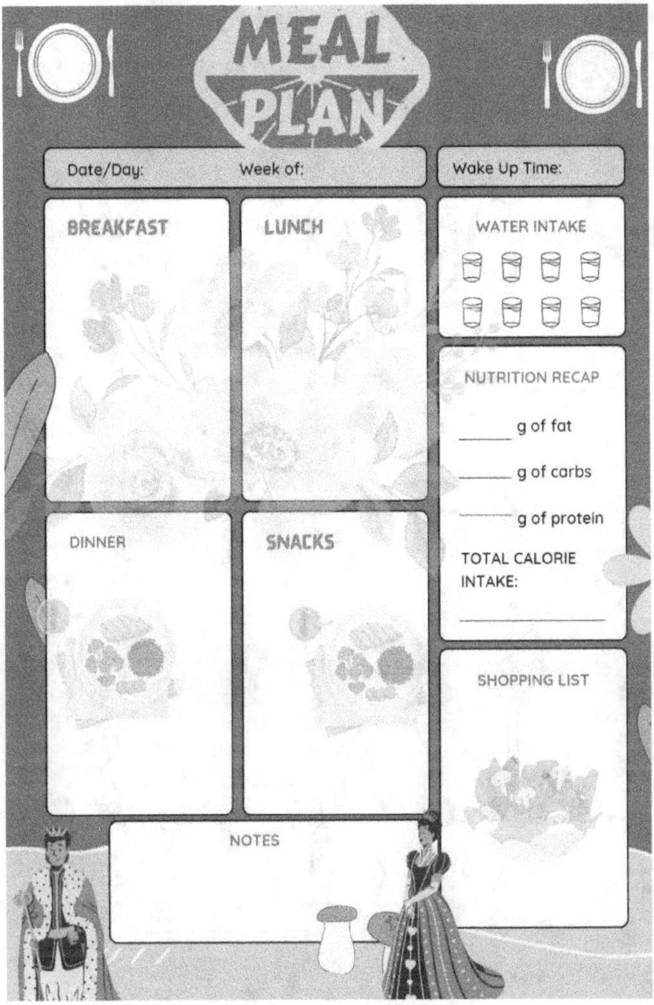

# MEAL PLAN

| Date/Day: | Week of: | Wake Up Time: |

## BREAKFAST

## LUNCH

### WATER INTAKE

### NUTRITION RECAP

________ g of fat

________ g of carbs

________ g of protein

TOTAL CALORIE INTAKE:

________________

## DINNER

## SNACKS

### SHOPPING LIST

### NOTES

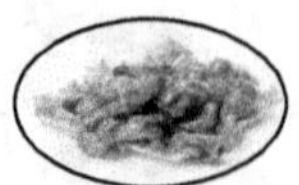
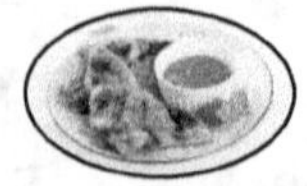
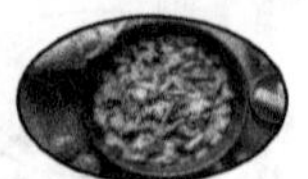

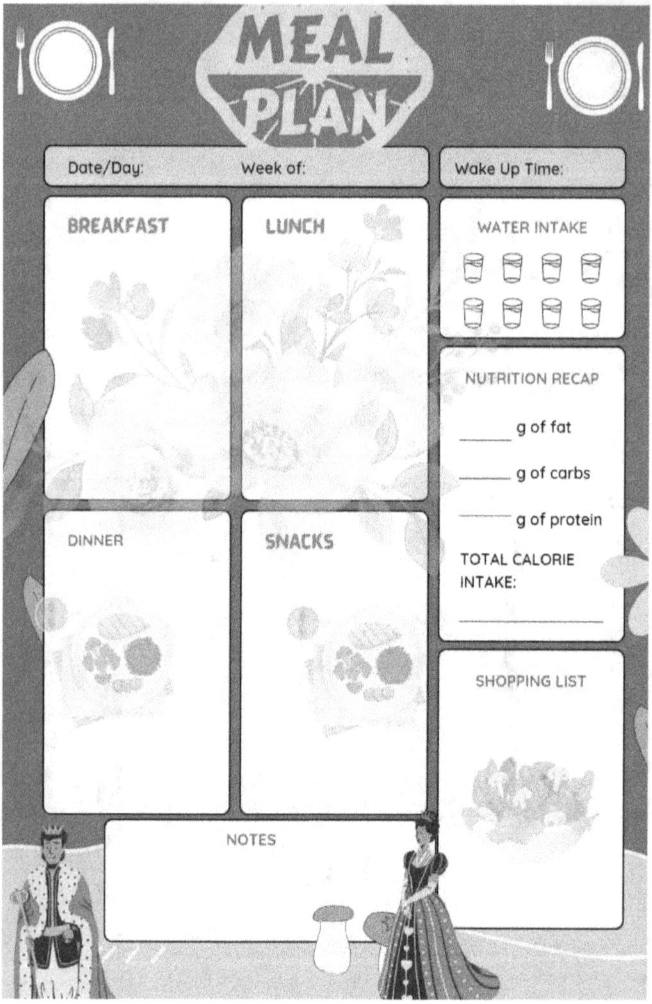

# MEAL PLAN

| Date/Day: | Week of: | Wake Up Time: |
| --- | --- | --- |

## BREAKFAST

## LUNCH

## WATER INTAKE

## NUTRITION RECAP

_______ g of fat

_______ g of carbs

_______ g of protein

TOTAL CALORIE INTAKE:

________________

## DINNER

## SNACKS

## SHOPPING LIST

## NOTES

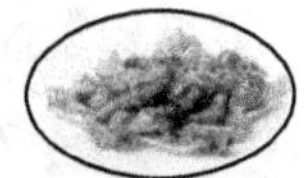 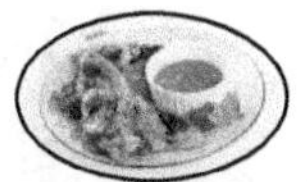 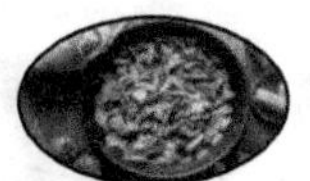

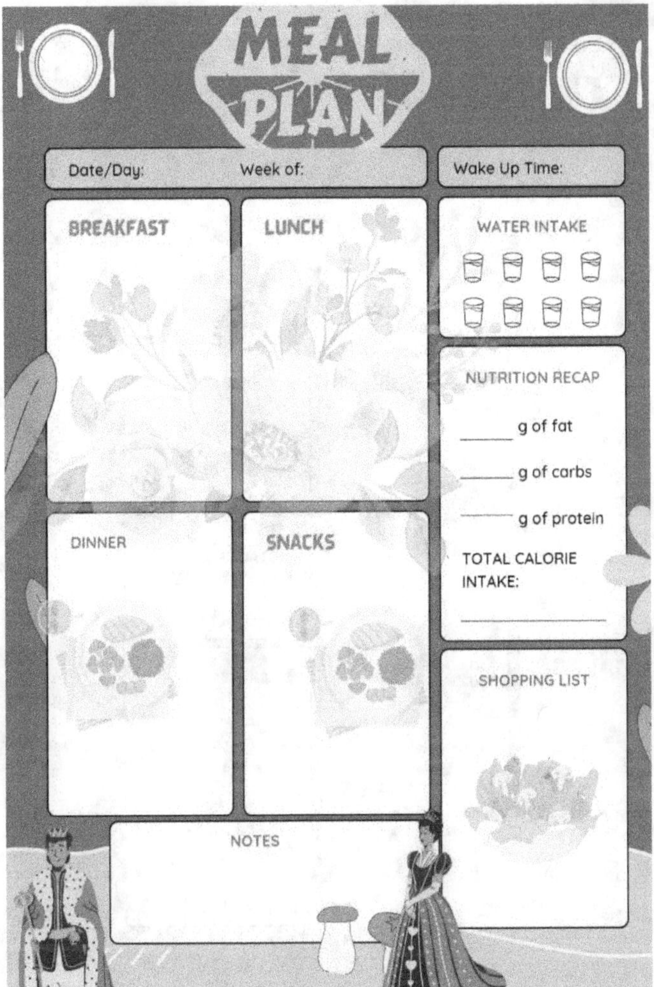

# MEAL PLAN

| Date/Day: | Week of: | Wake Up Time: |

## BREAKFAST

## LUNCH

## WATER INTAKE

## NUTRITION RECAP

_______ g of fat

_______ g of carbs

_______ g of protein

TOTAL CALORIE INTAKE:

_______________

## DINNER

## SNACKS

## SHOPPING LIST

## NOTES

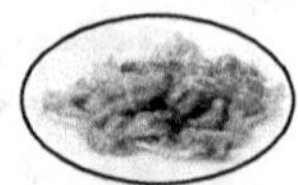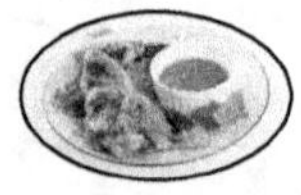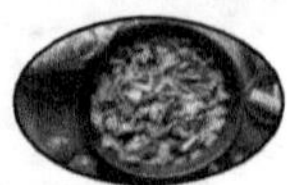

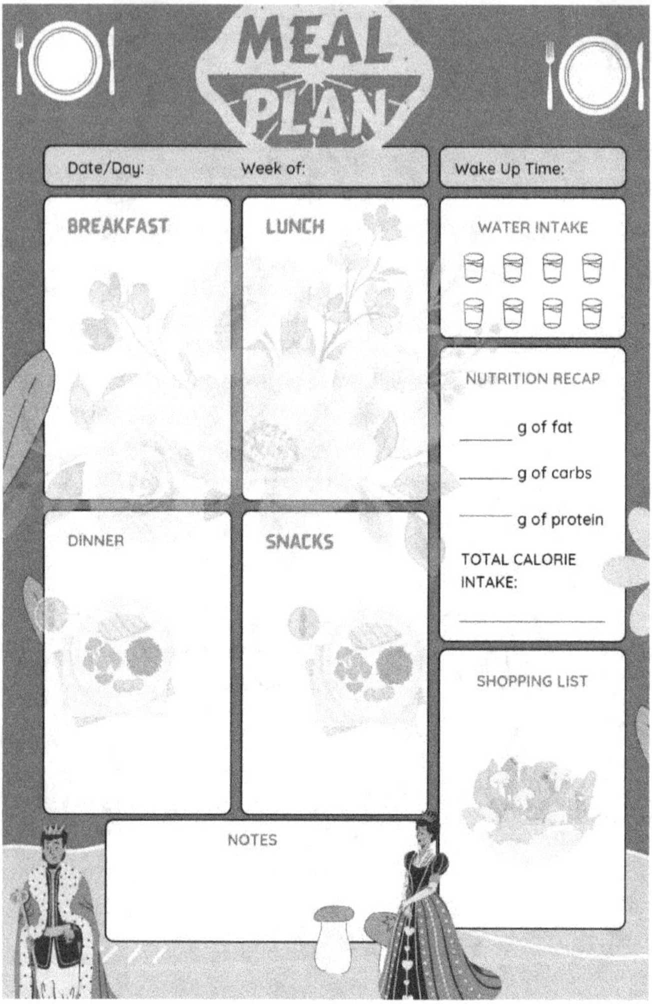

# MEAL PLAN

| Date/Day: | Week of: | Wake Up Time: |

## BREAKFAST

## LUNCH

### WATER INTAKE

### NUTRITION RECAP

_______ g of fat

_______ g of carbs

_______ g of protein

TOTAL CALORIE INTAKE:

_______________

## DINNER

## SNACKS

### SHOPPING LIST

### NOTES

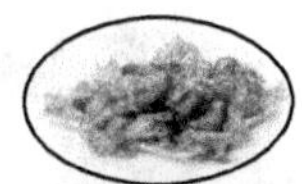 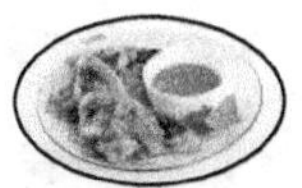 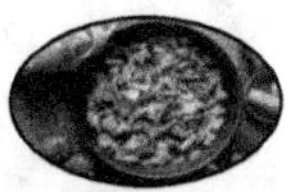

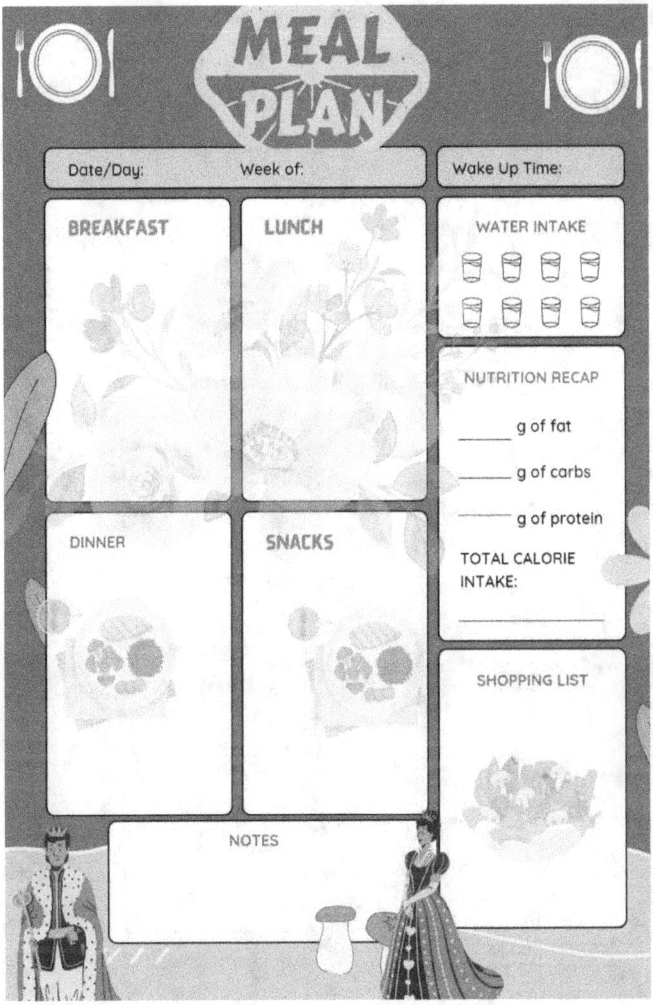

# MEAL PLAN

| Date/Day: | Week of: | Wake Up Time: |
| --- | --- | --- |

## BREAKFAST

## LUNCH

## WATER INTAKE

## NUTRITION RECAP

_______ g of fat

_______ g of carbs

_______ g of protein

TOTAL CALORIE INTAKE:

_______________

## DINNER

## SNACKS

## SHOPPING LIST

## NOTES

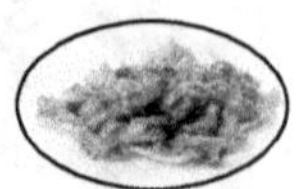 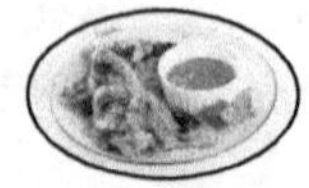 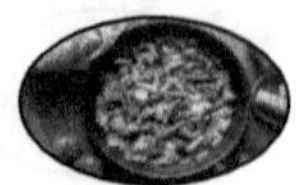

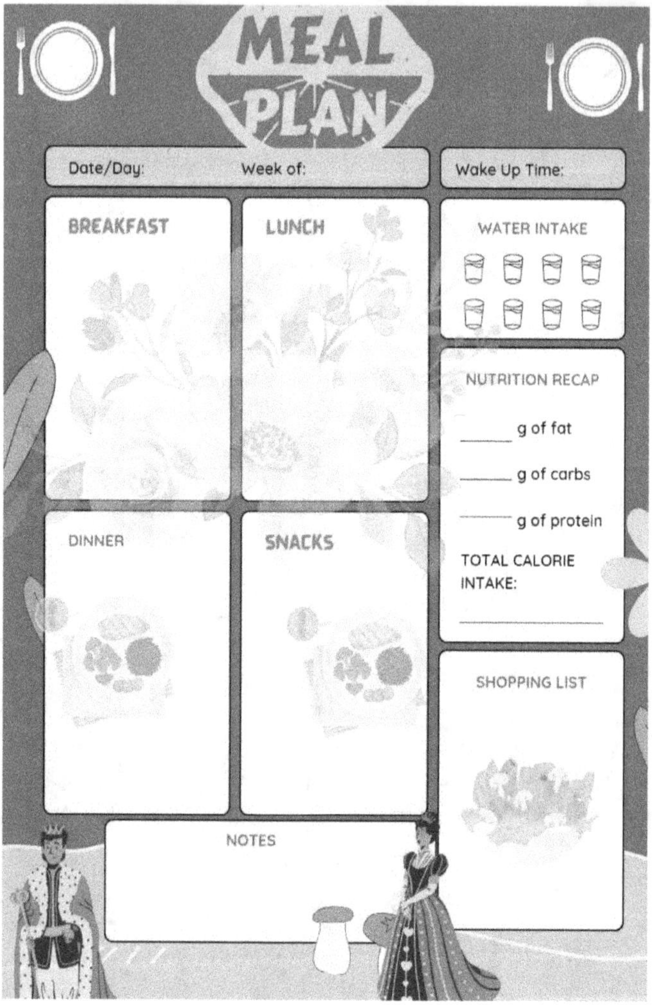

# MEAL PLAN

| Date/Day: | Week of: | Wake Up Time: |
| --- | --- | --- |

## BREAKFAST

## LUNCH

### WATER INTAKE

### NUTRITION RECAP

__________ g of fat

__________ g of carbs

__________ g of protein

**TOTAL CALORIE INTAKE:**

__________

## DINNER

## SNACKS

### SHOPPING LIST

### NOTES

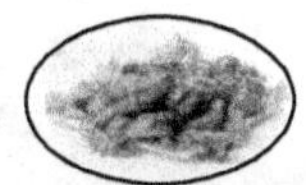 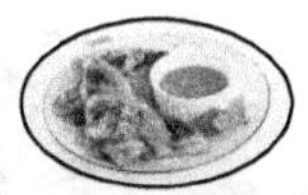 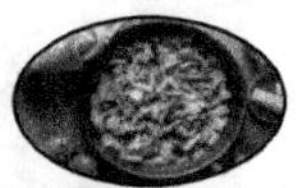

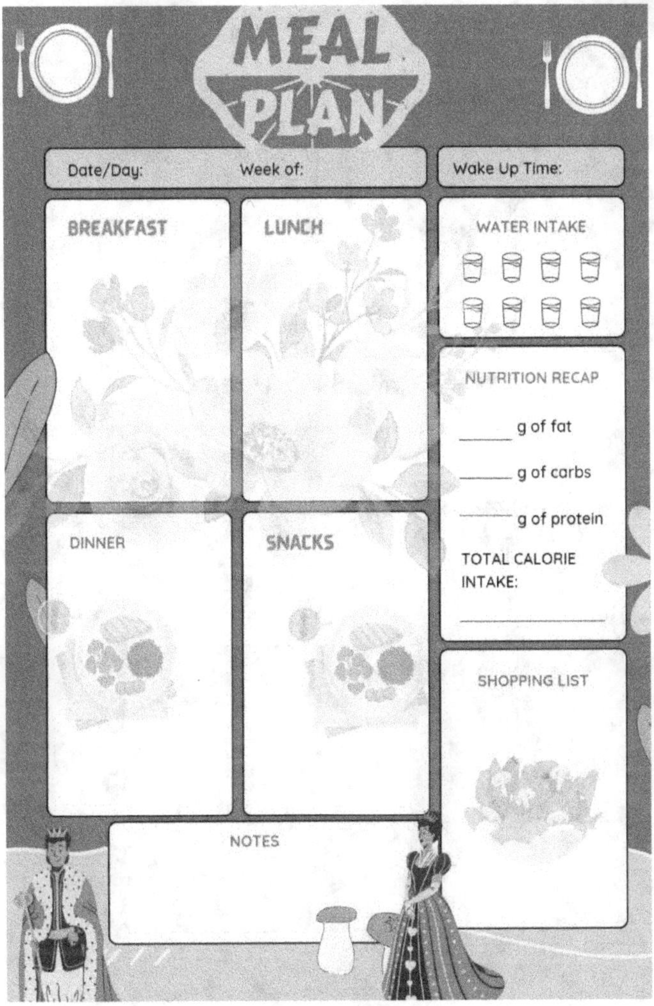

# MEAL PLAN

| Date/Day: | Week of: | Wake Up Time: |

## BREAKFAST

## LUNCH

### WATER INTAKE

### NUTRITION RECAP

________ g of fat

________ g of carbs

________ g of protein

TOTAL CALORIE INTAKE:

________________

## DINNER

## SNACKS

### SHOPPING LIST

### NOTES

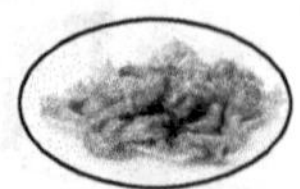 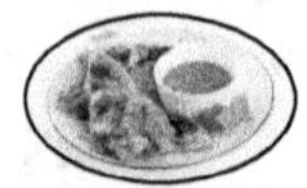 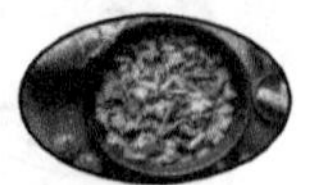

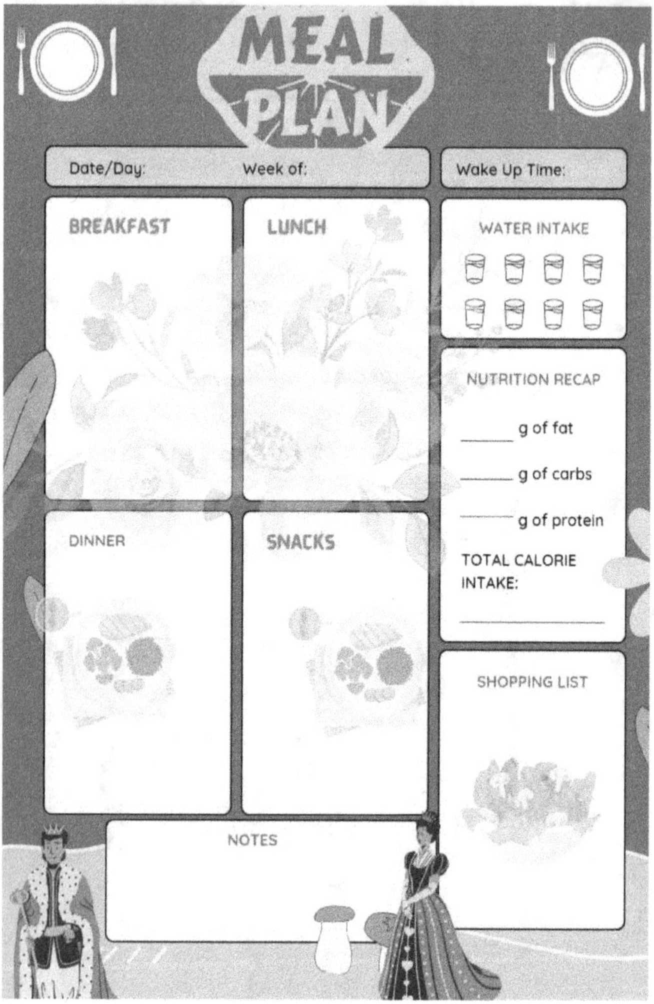

# MEAL PLAN

Date/Day: | Week of: | Wake Up Time:

## BREAKFAST

## LUNCH

## WATER INTAKE

## NUTRITION RECAP

__________ g of fat

__________ g of carbs

__________ g of protein

TOTAL CALORIE INTAKE:

__________

## DINNER

## SNACKS

## SHOPPING LIST

## NOTES

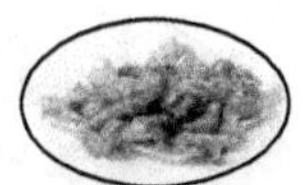 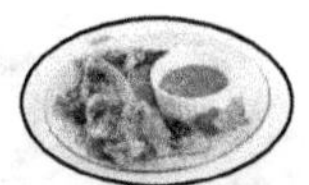 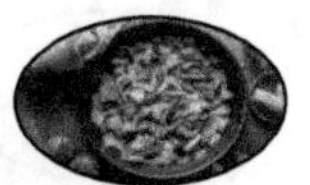

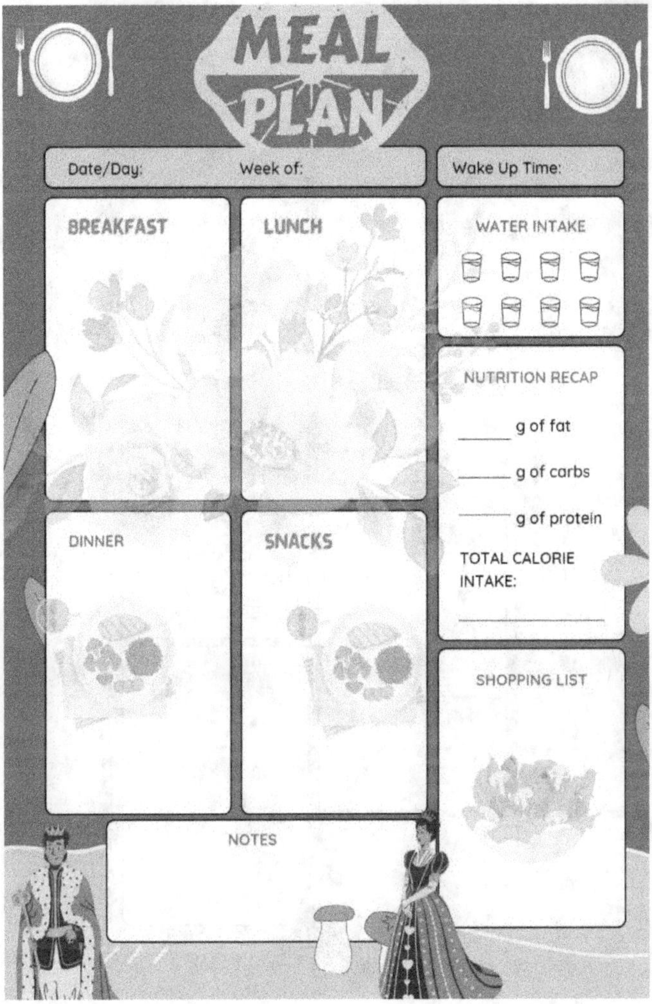

# MEAL PLAN

| Date/Day: | Week of: | Wake Up Time: |

## BREAKFAST

## LUNCH

### WATER INTAKE

### NUTRITION RECAP

_______ g of fat

_______ g of carbs

_______ g of protein

**TOTAL CALORIE INTAKE:**

_______________

## DINNER

## SNACKS

### SHOPPING LIST

### NOTES

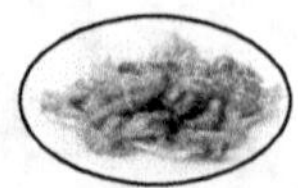 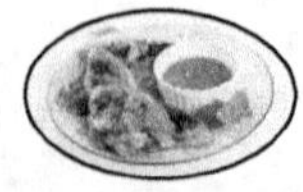 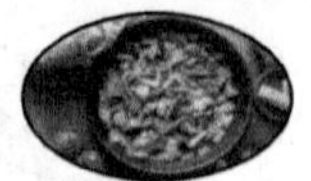

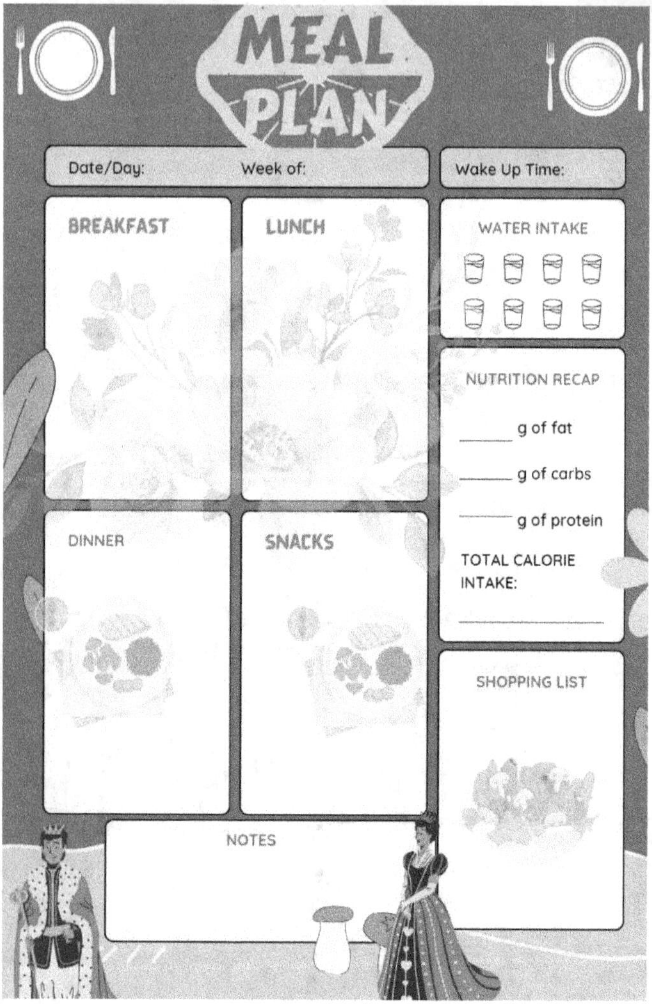

# MEAL PLAN

| Date/Day: | Week of: | Wake Up Time: |

## BREAKFAST

## LUNCH

### WATER INTAKE

### NUTRITION RECAP

________ g of fat

________ g of carbs

________ g of protein

TOTAL CALORIE INTAKE:

________________

## DINNER

## SNACKS

### SHOPPING LIST

## NOTES

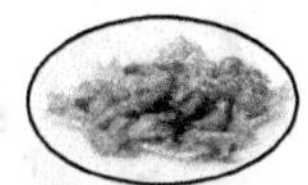 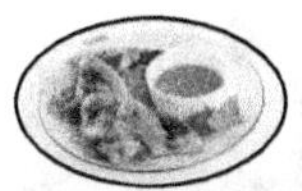 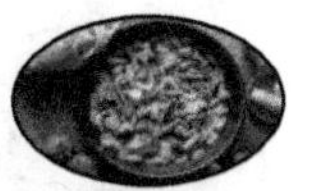

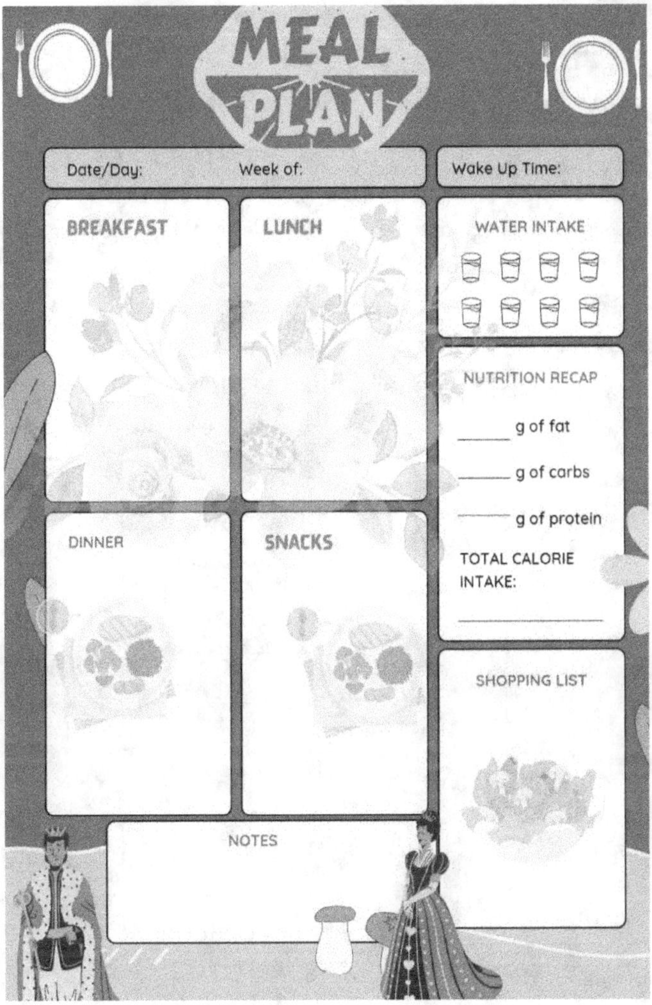

# MEAL PLAN

| Date/Day: | Week of: | Wake Up Time: |

## BREAKFAST

## LUNCH

### WATER INTAKE

### NUTRITION RECAP

______ g of fat

______ g of carbs

______ g of protein

TOTAL CALORIE INTAKE:

______

### DINNER

### SNACKS

### SHOPPING LIST

### NOTES

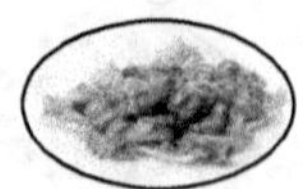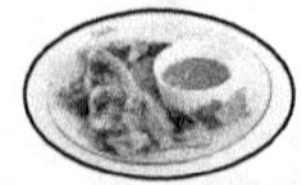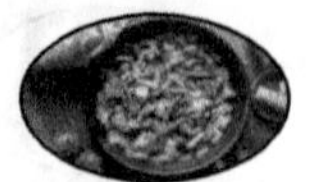

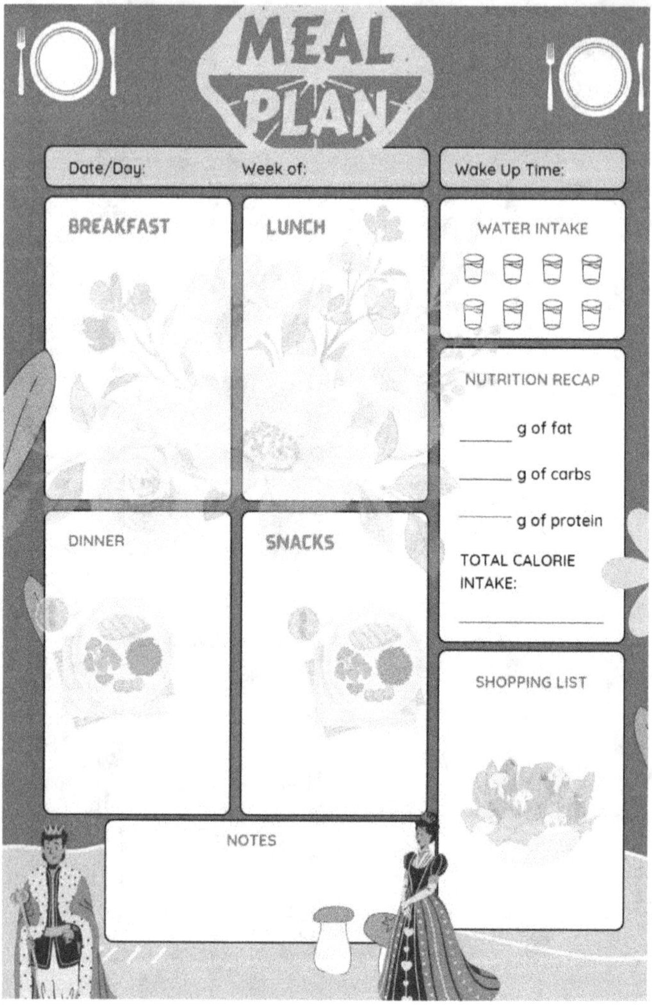

# MEAL PLAN

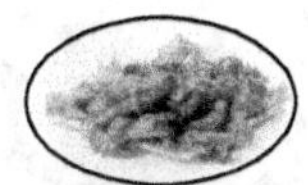 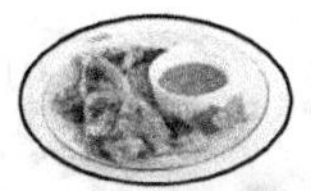 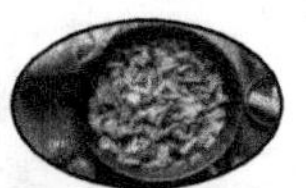

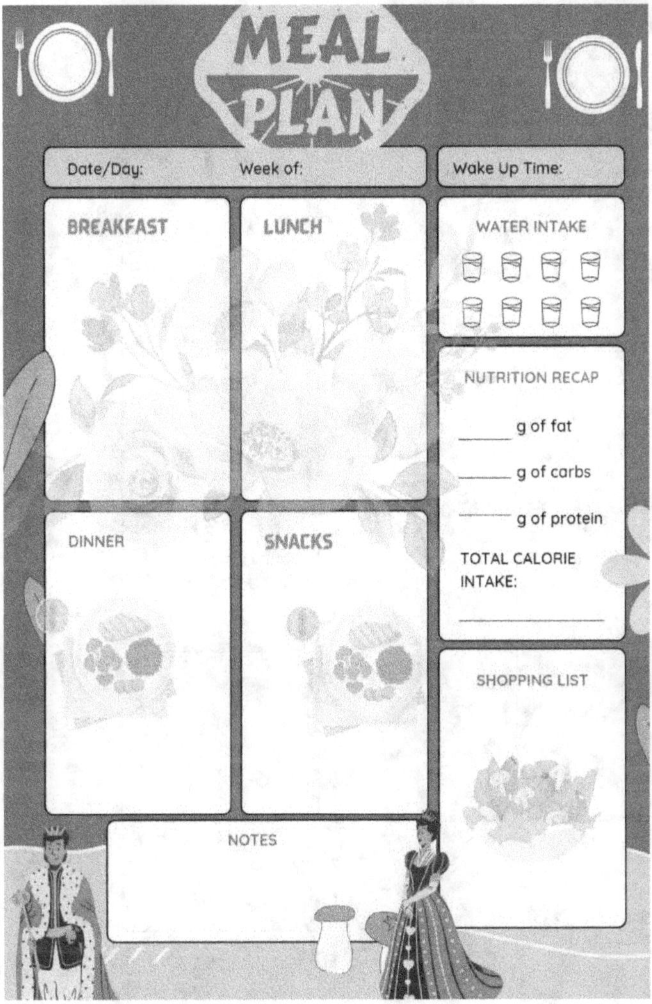

# MEAL PLAN

| Date/Day: | Week of: | Wake Up Time: |

## BREAKFAST

## LUNCH

### WATER INTAKE

### NUTRITION RECAP

_______ g of fat

_______ g of carbs

_______ g of protein

TOTAL CALORIE INTAKE:

_______________

## DINNER

## SNACKS

### SHOPPING LIST

### NOTES

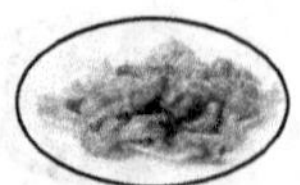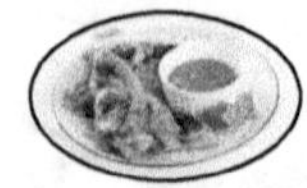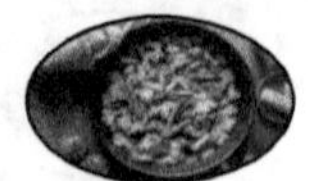

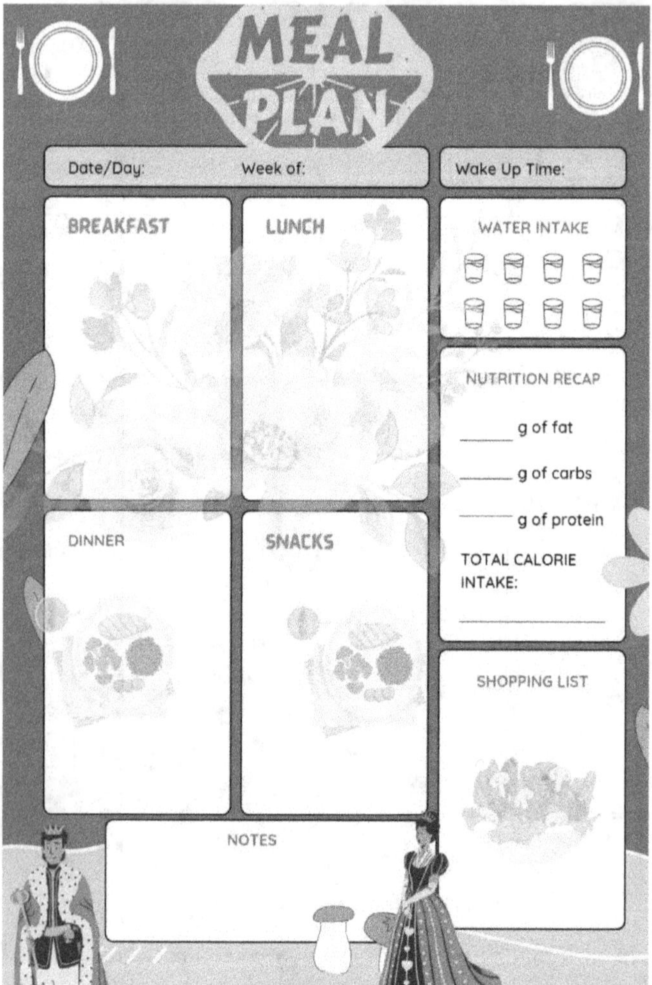

# MEAL PLAN

| Date/Day: | Week of: | Wake Up Time: |

## BREAKFAST

## LUNCH

### WATER INTAKE

### NUTRITION RECAP

________ g of fat

________ g of carbs

________ g of protein

**TOTAL CALORIE INTAKE:**

________

## DINNER

## SNACKS

### SHOPPING LIST

### NOTES